The Theory and Science of Basketball

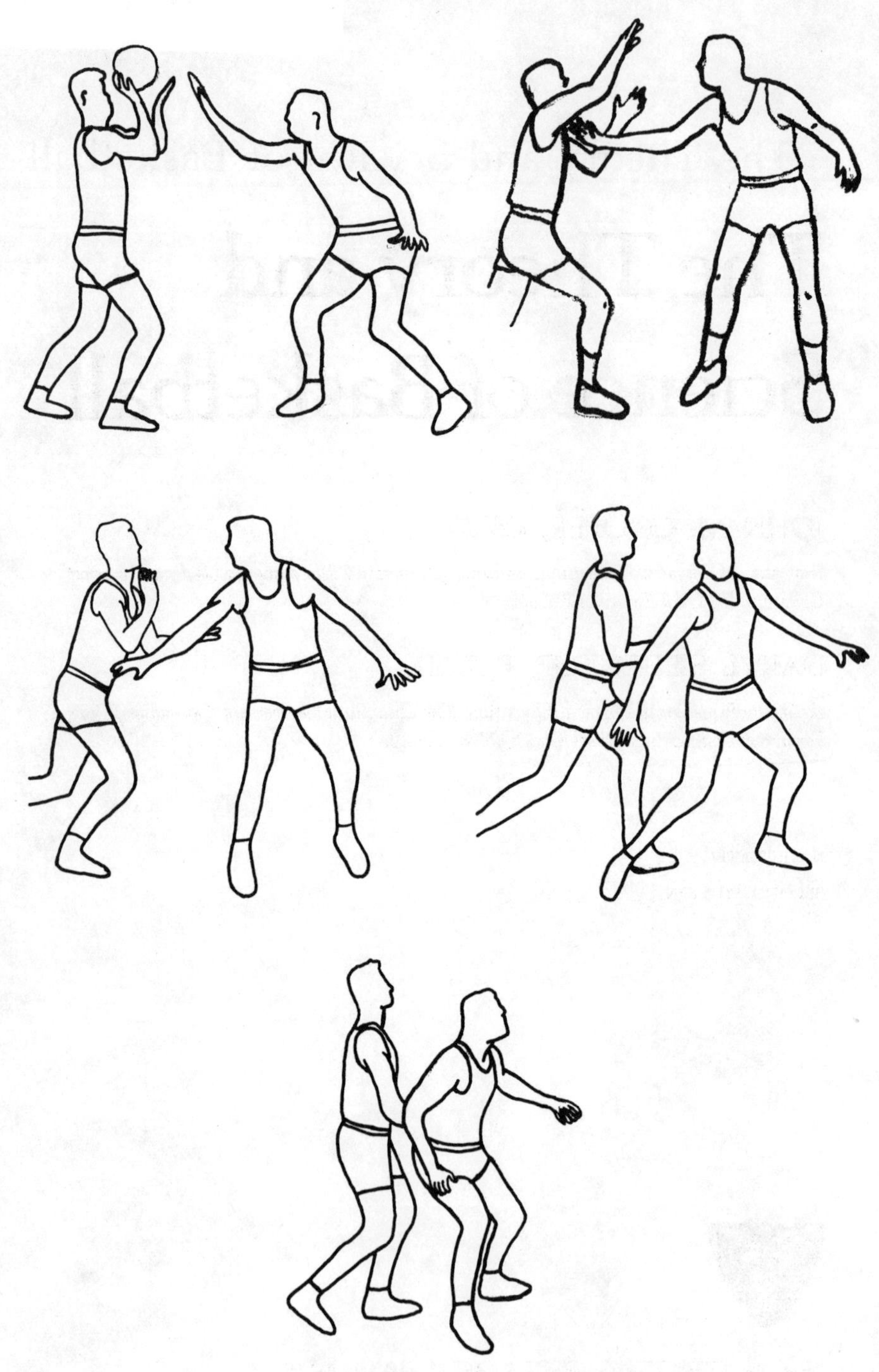

The Theory and Science of Basketball

JOHN M. COOPER, Ed. D.

Professor of Physical Education, Indiana University, Bloomington, Indiana, Former College and AAU Basketball Coach

DARYL SIEDENTOP, P. E. D.

Associate Professor of Physical Education, The Ohio State University, Columbus, Ohio, Former Assistant Basketball Coach, Hope College

ILLUSTRATED

SECOND EDITION

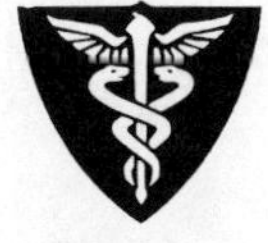

LEA & FEBIGER · PHILADELPHIA · 1975

Health Education, Physical Education, and Recreation Series

RUTH ABERNATHY, PH.D., EDITORIAL ADVISER
Professor Emeritus
School of Physical and Health Education,
University of Washington, Seattle, Washington, 98105

Library of Congress Cataloging in Publication Data

Cooper, John Miller, 1912–
The theory and science of basketball.

(Health education, physical education, and recreation series)
Bibliography: p.
1. Basketball. I. Siedentop, Daryl, joint author. II. Title.
GV885.C624 1975 796.32'32 74-4376
ISBN 0-8121-0502-8

First Edition, 1969
Reprinted, 1970
Second Edition, 1975

Published in Great Britain by Henry Kimpton Publishers, London
PRINTED IN THE UNITED STATES OF AMERICA

to our families
for their patience and forebearance

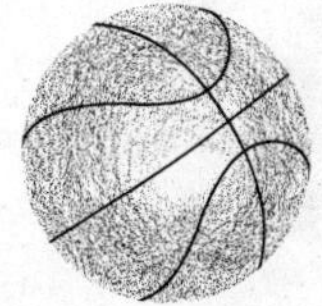

Foreword

This second edition upgrades and updates the fine basketball book written by Cooper and Siedentop. This book has proved to be one of the few really outstanding and lasting contributions made to the literature in the field of basketball.

It appears that a repeat of what was previously written about the authors with some updating needs to be done in this edition. Dr. John M. Cooper brings impressive credentials to the task of writing on the subject of basketball. For over thirty years he has been a close student of the game, as a player, coach, teacher, and consultant. This broad view is combined with an abiding dedication to the game of basketball and those who play and coach it. Recently, he and his students at Indiana University, where he is now located, have been doing research in some of the finer details of the game never yet investigated. One coach from a large university told me that he was so fascinated by the first edition when he received it, he sat up all night reading it. The second edition is equally irresistible to the basketball-minded individual.

Dr. Cooper was an extraordinary high school player, once scoring 500 points in one season. Later, he was an excellent college player at the University of Missouri where he is now given credit as being the first college player actually to use the jump shot as a primary offensive weapon. This fact perhaps indicates his willingness to experiment with new ideas and to test their practical consequences for increased skill in basketball performance. During his playing career at Missouri, he is credited with scoring approximately 47 percent of his team's points in a single year. This is the highest percentage recorded in the history of the Big Eight Conference, exceeding such all-time greats as Clyde Lovellett and Wilt Chamberlain.

Prior to going to the University of Southern California, he was a successful high school and college coach. Concurrently with fulfilling his responsibilities at U.S.C. he coached the Southern California AAU champions for two years.

During his years as a teacher he has had an opportunity to exert an influence over many young and aspiring basketball coaches. It was in just such a situation that my long and close association with him began at the University of Southern California where he was on the Physical Education staff for twenty-one years. As a teacher he was able to bring the application of scientific evidence down to the practical level and apply it to the every day problems that coaches face in developing players. His was a lasting influence on me, as well as on other students such as Bill Sharman and Tex Winter. He was never too busy to sit down and discuss basketball problems with his students and try to find ways to improve old methods and create new ones.

This book is a reflection of his excellent teaching. He brings to it the same experience and practicality that made his classroom an exciting place to be. He is an experienced writer, which in itself makes this book an oddity among the many books in print on the subject of basketball. He expresses his basic ideas with clarity and with a minimum of extraneous words. The principles approach utilized in the book should be a major contribution to the development of sports literature. The principles reflect, in a practical way, a professional lifetime spent in the scientific study of movement skills in general and basketball skills in particular.

Daryl Siedentop, the co-author, has recently been engaged in coaching basketball at the college level. Also, since the publication of the first edition, he has become an outstanding young scholar in several fields of endeavor, yet still maintaining his deep and inquisitive interest in basketball. He was engaged so that the ideas expressed herein would be relevant to the day-to-day problems that a basketball coach faces in the competitive world in which the game is pursued today. Daryl Siedentop played on Hope College basketball teams from 1956–1960. During this four-year period, the Hope teams compiled a fantastic 73–15 record, won four Michigan Intercollegiate Athletic Association championships, and made two trips to the NCAA college division tournament. Daryl joined his college tutor, Coach Russ DeVette, as an assistant immediately following his graduation. As a player and a coach, Daryl was a part of a winning tradition at Hope College that could boast of nine conference championships in eleven years.

In addition several young and successful coaches have reviewed the manuscript for its correctness of terminology and elucidation of ideas. Their suggestions are included.

It gives me a great pleasure to recommend this revised book to all coaches and students of the game of basketball. It contains valuable information that will be an excellent book to use in basketball theory classes for undergraduate and graduate students who aspire to be successful coaches.

Bob Boyd
Head Basketball Coach
University of Southern California
Los Angeles

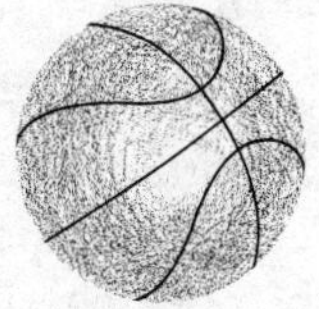

Preface

We have retained in this second edition most of the unique features of the first edition. We still believe we can discuss the various aspects of the game with more than reasonable objectivity since we are not currently engaged in coaching basketball. The first of these features is that we do not advocate the use of any one "system" of basketball. The use of any one offense in preference to any other or any one defense over another is not presented. Rather, an attempt is made to present a comprehensive picture of the advantages and disadvantages (their strengths and weaknesses) of the major current offensive and defensive systems.

We have updated some portions and in several instances completely rewritten certain sections. Several terms have been changed to bring the contents in line with the latest basketball terminology.

The development approach has been updated and retained in the presentation of the material. That is, an attempt is made to present suggestions and steps that the coach may utilize in the development of his own offensive and defensive systems. To accomplish this task, the principles approach to the subject matter of basketball is used. Wherever possible, specific principles are suggested that can be used to form the foundation upon which a coach may build his own offensive and defensive system that would be in keeping with his understanding of and his philosophical concepts related to the game. For these reasons, it is thought that this book might be particularly suited for use by students in the basketball theory classes at the undergraduate and graduate levels in the colleges and universities, as well as for all coaches of basketball at every level.

The second major feature of this book is the use of knowledge generated from the scientific analysis of human movement and the scientific study of the learning process. This is a true unique feature. This information is not presented using scientific terminology. That would confuse rather than clarify the problems of coaching. Rather the knowledge of the authors' scientific disciplines is taken and translated into workable suggestions for coaching. Modern coaches in every sport are making better use of the results of research. This is true both for results from biomechanics (the science of human movement and behavioral psychology (the science of human behavior). Track coaches, swimming coaches, and football coaches are all beginning to be more aware that they can improve performance by utilizing principles and findings derived from scientific research. The inclusion in this text of principles derived from research has, it is hoped, been made meaningful. It is believed that such principles are crucial to a thorough understanding of the topic under discussion. It would serve no purpose to insert scientifically based suggestions that were not useful in the real world of coaching. Scientific information is of little value to basketball coaches if it does not help them to develop players who are more highly skilled and teams that have a better chance of winning games. The motivation for presenting these principles is not for the purpose of impressing coaches with the scientific expertise of the authors. Indeed, it has been the authors' experience that most coaches have a "show me" attitude toward scientists and academicians. This skepticism is healthy. The purpose here has been to take what is useful and put it to service by passing it on to those who can best use it.

Originally we planned to have a young successful woman coach present her ideas in this edition. After writing down some concepts to be included she and her fellow coaches suggested that all that was needed was to state "skill is skill" and is not restricted to sex. We have done as she and they advised.

The organizational plan used here is not unique and was not replaced in this edition. Indeed, it seems to represent the consensus of many people concerning the best order of presentation to use in studying about the game of basketball. However, there are several topics included in each major division that are unusual, some of which we have updated and we have completely rewritten two sections.

In Chapter 1, The Game of Basketball, the sections on Principles of Learning and Predictions for the Future are examples of this uniqueness. It also appeared to be a good procedure to present the individual and team aspects of basketball separately. Thus, these latter form the second and third parts of the book.

Chapter 2, Individual Fundamentals, contains most of the practically applied scientific principles.

Chapter 3, Formation of Offensive and Defensive Systems, basically reflects the broad comprehensive approach taken in the presentation of the material. No single system of play is advocated over another. Rather, an attempt is made realistically to assess and offer advice about problems and situations that the coach will face in selecting and developing offensive and defensive systems.

In Chapter 4, Administration, an attempt is made to relate the practical importance of the effective accomplishment of administrative tasks to the total success of the basketball program. It may be stated that in the final analysis the use of good administrative techniques should help the coach to be successful in his work as a basketball coach.

Chapter 5, The Basketball Class in Physical Education, is included under the assumption that most high school and many college basketball coaches in the United States are also involved (directly or indirectly) in the teaching of physical education classes or in the training of future coaches and teachers. It is hoped that the ideas presented here will be of value to these teachers.

Finally, since the entire world is rapidly moving toward a standard set of international rules, we have included a summary of the differences between the collegiate and international rules. This will be found at the end of the book.

We acknowledge the contributions that we have received from many coaches and students of the game of basketball. Also, we are very appreciative of the specific suggestions given us by a recent fine player, Douglas Ash, formerly of Hanover College. We gratefully acknowledge the typing of the manuscript done by Charlianna Cooper.

JOHN M. COOPER
Bloomington, Indiana

DARYL SIEDENTOP
Columbus, Ohio

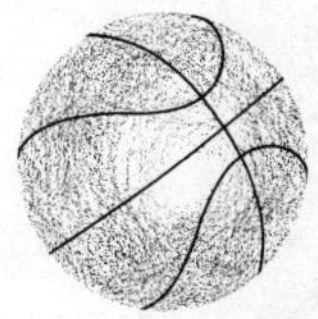

Contents

The Theory and Science of Basketball

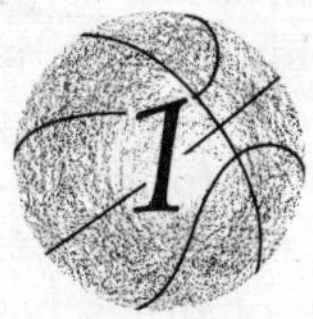

The Game of Basketball

Philosophy of Coaching

Coaches usually state that one of the primary objectives in coaching basketball is to motivate the players to attempt to win. In the final analysis then, their philosophy of coaching basketball is embodied in this concept. Thus, such conceived philosophy of coaching is related in a great measure to the answer given to the question: "How far am I willing to go to win games?"

Nobody actively involved in sports and coaching disagrees with the competitive concept of striving to win. Indeed, the very nature of games makes vital and necessary the desire to compete and win. To do less does dishonor both to the game and to the opponent. On the other hand, we know of almost no coach who would "go to any lengths" in order to secure a victory, at least not if he takes seriously into consideration what might occur if he pursued winning with no restraints being placed on him. A practicing philosophy of coaching is best seen in the methods a coach is willing to utilize in order to win. It is fine to wax eloquent at banquet speeches, but the real test of a philosophy of coaching is found in how a coach treats his players, the demands he places on them, and the total context within which he pursues his goals in his basketball program. Some of the statements made in the subsequent pages will serve to bring into focus certain of our beliefs. No attempt has been made to cover all of the ethical and moral decisions that a coach makes in planning and implementing a basketball program. We hope a sufficient number of points is raised to provoke thought and discussion. Each coach must decide for himself what he believes and then he must act accordingly. It is hoped that what he says and what he does will reflect by his actions consistently with what he says he believes.

The coach, just to try to win, *should not jeopardize the health of any player on his team* in any way; neither his physical nor his mental health. The use of drugs to attempt to stimulate for greater performances and/or to allow players with serious injuries to perform are doubtful practices. The coach should not focus his attention just on the basketball game to the exclusion of all other aspects. The intake of drugs has not proved to be beneficial. In the case of physical injuries, the coach should rely entirely on a physician's recommendation based upon his personal examination of the injury as to whether to play a boy or not. *The problem of maintaining the proper mental-emotional well-being of each player is the responsibility of the coach,* not the physician. Therefore, he must deal with each individual player according to his needs. The coach acts as a reasonable and prudent protector of the player's mental health by treating him as a unique individual. In turn, he must demand the same respect from the players. It is obvious that, for good or bad, the coach is serving as a model for the players to emulate. If the coach is insensitive to the individual needs of his players, then this procedure is likely to become the standard pattern of behavior adopted for use by the members of his team.

Another aspect that should be mentioned is that the coach's relationship with and attitude toward the opposing team has an effect on his players. The coach should never make fun of the players on the other team. Nor should he ever single out an opposing player for abuse. It is also a bad practice for a coach to run up a high score on a weaker team by leaving in his best players for the entirety of the game. This is not only a display of bad manners, but it is poor strategy as the experience may tend to cause the regular players to be unprepared for tougher opponents whom they will come up against at a later date. Also, next year the opposing coach may have a team strong enough to turn the tables on him. The coach should be courteous and respectful to the opposing coach and players at all times. How friendly he is with the opposition is largely a matter of individual choice. It is generally recognized as good practice for the coach not to be overly friendly with the opposing players. On the other hand, when an obvious mistake has been made by the official, he need not be a "milk sop" type. The coach has the responsibility to point out gross officiating errors to the officials.

The coach's relationship to the spectators is also of importance in determining their response to him and his players. The coach should realize that his behavior during the game is a matter of public record. It can help influence the attitude of the crowd toward almost any aspect of the game. For example, a coach who is constantly up off the bench yelling at the officials and players will engender the same kind of behavior from the spectators, especially at home contests. The coach simply cannot overlook the fact that he is a representative of an educational institution, and that his behavior in public will be regarded in that context.

The coach also must deal with his players, firmly, individually, and fairly if he is to gain their respect and loyalty. In as far as it is possible, each boy must be treated in such a manner that he knows that equality is not just a byword. Also, the boys must understand that they, too, are representatives of a school and that their behavior before, during, and after the game will be considered as a reflection on that school. This point of view pertains to matters of personal appearance, behavior on the bench, behavior in public places such as in restaurants, and behavior on the bus traveling to and from the games. Mutual respect between the players and coach is the attainment of the ideal state of affairs.

Another important aspect to consider in this connection that is often overlooked is the behavior of the boys in the locker room. It is in the locker room more than anywhere else that a coach's beliefs could be best observed in action. While the coach should not as a rule "police" the locker room, the players must understand that certain standards of conduct must be upheld and that certain types of behavior will not be permitted in this environment.

Finally, the coach must keep in mind that he is an educator, and one who is in a unique position to have great influence on the values considered important by his players. If he neglects this obligation, he has not met his educational responsibility to help contribute to the growth and development of young women and men.

Comparison of Play Now with That of the Past

The game of basketball had its origin at Springfield, Massachusetts, at the International YMCA training school, in 1891. It is important to remember that Dr. James Naismith, the inventor of the game, was seeking a means, as an instructor at the school, to interest his class of business men in physical exercise. The men were disinterested in mass participation in calisthenics and exercises. Many innovations of known games and drills were tried but all failed to keep the lasting interest of the group.

Finally, almost in desperation, Naismith invented a game which combined some elements of soccer, and rugby football into a new game. The new game was to involve no personal contact among players and to make use of an elevated goal. One of the men named the game at the very first experience with it and it held their interest from the start. From this beginning, the game spread so rapidly that by 1920 it had become a national pastime.

The first basket was funnel-shaped and as consequence gave rise to the development of a net tailored to this shape. The iron rim was the only portion of the goal apparatus used after the abandonment of the so-called "peach" basket. In the 20's and 30's string, cloth and leather nets were introduced (later even wide steel mesh was experimented with) and tried out with the string or cord net becoming the standard equipment that was officially adopted. The rim was once fastened flush against the back board (made of wood), then later projected out from the board (standard 15 cm). The glass board was used earlier in a few gymnasiums, but discarded for a while but now universally adopted.

It is also important to remember that the rules, position of players, and methods of play used in soccer and football form the basis for the rules and conduct of play selected for the game of basketball. Furthermore, it should be stated that many of the players who participated in the first game were well grounded in the nomenclature and fundamentals of soccer and rugby football. Consequently, the formation first used and the names applied to the players' positions, etc., reveal that they were copied from these games. The use of a basket and the elimination of running with the ball aspects were in a sense modifications of these previously mentioned games. While it was purposely invented, its acceptance was predicated on the idea that it must be liked and enjoyed before being adopted.

The question is often asked, "Why do people like to toss a basketball at the basket?" Because, first it is believed that almost anyone can perform (and challenge) to see if and how many goals can be made. Some success usually occurs in shooting at the basket no matter how limited the experience has been. Practically all the action of the teams and players is seen and understood by observers. These are among the many reasons it is believed that basketball grew so rapidly in popularity as a sport for participants and spectators.

The main principles of play and major governing rules as conceived at the time of the invention are the foundation upon which the game operates today. Naismith* believed that the main difference in the way the game is played today in comparison with early days resides in the increased skill of the modern players. This change in ability has been brought about because the moves made by top players are easily seen and soon copied by others. The maneuvers of the college, AAU and professional players today are those that will be used tomorrow by the high school player. Consequently, progress in ability was and is inevitable.

The contribution of the coaches to the game in the past has been mostly in the realm of team play and court discipline and the ability to recognize

*Naismith, James: *Basketball*, Association Press, New York, 1941.

the value of new moves that players invent and to install these moves into a consistent pattern of play. It is significant to note that most of the improvement in skill per se has been done by the players themselves in response to the opponent, facilities or general environment, and/or because of their own physical abilities or limitations. Even in "horsing around" during the off season new ideas arose and new skills were thus developed. It may be said that basketball offered the opportunity for the players to use originality and ingenuity in developing new moves and in perfecting old ones.

A comparison of the play now with that of yesterday may offer an inspiration to present players to go on to make even greater contributions toward the future development of the game. It may help the young player or coach to be more aware of the opportunities that are available to develop and utilize new skills and techniques. It may also help to increase a historical appreciation for the "American" game of basketball.

We have experienced many of the styles and maneuvers mentioned in these pages. Some were heard of from players and coaches having had experience with the game previously. Others were discovered on the printed page of old basketball books and are now told in this historical account.

By 1896, after the game had undergone some trial, the first players were called by position, left forward, right forward, left center, right center, left back, right back, and goalie* again giving evidence to the influence of the game of soccer and football. By 1897 some positions were eliminated and the five positions used today were adopted.†

The manner of team play even several years after its origin still showed the soccer influence. During the years of 1910 to 1923 each team had a standing and running guard and a standing and running forward along with a center. The standing guard was used primarily as a defensive player similar to that of a goalie in soccer. The running guard helped on defense and went into the offensive territory to aid the forwards in scoring. He was usually smaller and quicker than the standing guard.

The standing forward was used primarily on offense to do the scoring and remained mostly in offensive territory. The running forward often moved the length of the court helping not only in scoring, but in passing the ball to the standing forward. All the other players were primarily involved in passing the ball directly or indirectly to the forwards, usually the standing forward. Since one player in these early days attempted all free throws that his team was awarded, the standing forward often was designated as the player to attempt these "charity tosses." This condition

*Naismith, James: Op. Cit. p. 95.
†Naismith, James: Op. Cit. p. 73.

prevailed until the 1923–24 season when the present rule, stating that a player against whom the foul was committed must attempt the free throw, was put into effect.* This rule gave the opportunity to all players to score if fouled. Its effect was the beginning of the gradual change for all players to become offensively minded.

The center at first did little more than jump at the center circle and serve as a safety valve for teammates to pass to if they could not pass the ball to the forwards. He sometimes played as a forward on offense, but usually he just aided and abetted the other players as a sort of somewhat silent partner. It was many years before the center became a key player in the game.

The play, from its origin until the early thirties, was considerably slower than the fire brand style used by many teams today. Scores were much lower than today because the play was for the most part much more deliberate. (There was also less playing time in a game because of the methods now used in stopping the clock after an infraction, etc.) The following changes helped to speed up the play in the game:

(1) The 1932–33 rules required that a team gaining possession of the ball in its own back court must advance the ball over the center line within ten seconds;

(2) Starting with the 1935–36 season the rules stated that after a successful free throw resulting from a personal foul the ball was put in play from out-of-bounds under the basket;

(3) In 1937–38, the center jump after a successful field goal was eliminated.

The standing forward (or sleeper as he could be called today), in the early days, received long passes the length of the floor, but he was usually flanked by the standing guard who seldom advanced beyond the center of the court toward his own basket. Consequently, the standing guard rarely shot the ball at the basket. The standing forward on the other hand was the team's top scorer and was fed the ball for scoring chances at every opportunity. Since there was no penalty for the time consumed in advancing the ball toward the offensive goal, most players passed the ball in a very deliberate manner from teammate to teammate as the ball was moved toward their own basket. If a player on a team scored a basket, the ball was put in play by the two centers jumping in the center of the court. This also tended to slow down the pace. Also, very few of the players were as offensively minded as they are today. Even the standing forward would usually attempt only six to eight shots at the basket during a game, with the rest of the players averaging zero to three attempts per game. The standing guard often made no attempt to score.

*Spaulding Basketball Rules, 1923–24.

From the year 1902 to 1914 basketball was played under so many different sets of rules it is difficult to determine what progress was actually made in standardizing them. The play was extremely rough because it was not made clear to the players to whom the ball should be awarded when it went out-of-bounds. Usually the first player to control it could throw it in. The gymnasiums having a running track in the balcony around the court were the scene of fights and melee when the ball missed the backboard and fell on to the elevated running track. All ten players sometimes ran after the ball to get it to put it in play.* The officials during this period seldom disqualified a player for excessive fouling or rough play.

The term "cage game" was named for the cage-like enclosure used for a court in some sections of the United States. The court was surrounded by wire or a net and no matter where the ball was located it was not out-of-bounds. Sometimes spectators became so excited and partisan that if an opposing player's hand accidentally went through the wire or net as he fell against it, he might find that his hand was rapped with a parasol or some object wielded by a spectator. Players used the wall as a target and they threw the ball against it on one side and retrieved it sometimes themselves on the opposite side. The ceiling was not out-of-bounds and where it was low, (many ceilings were about 14 feet high thus causing the player attempting a long shot to shoot directly at the basket) the ball could be bounced off of it into the basket. Players often "climbed" the wall near the basket when shooting short shots. "Dunking" the ball through the basket was occasionally done from a position off the wall. However, it was usually economically unsound to do so because often the goal was bent out of shape.

Also, many small schools during the twenties had only an outdoor court. Consequently, shots taken from long range were rare because of the effect of the wind. Some schools played basketball only during an outdoor season.

Since most high schools in many sections of the country before World War I (and even a few years after) did not have a school gymnasium, sometimes town halls and public meeting places were converted into basketball courts. Many of these buildings were supported by pillars located in rows throughout the structure including the playing court. The players adapted their play to make use of these obstructions. Also, the day of the cement floors, low ceilings and poor lighting, etc., spawned a careful player and caused team moves to be developed that were necessarily of a cautious nature. However, this era, 1910–25, added to the increase in player and team skill in the realm of good close-to-the-basket shooting and execution of quick, short passes used by the offensive team to penetrate tight defenses.

*Sempert, Dean: *Major Rule Changes in Men's Basketball from 1902 to 1954,* unpublished project, University of Southern California, Los Angeles, 1954, p. 15.

In certain cold regions of the country the buildings in which the indoor court was located were often very small. The stove heating the building was frequently located on or near the playing court and caused players to resort to unusual techniques in attempting to avoid it. It has been reported that visiting players had to play with one eye focused on the stove and one on the closest opponent, else they might find that they would be pushed into it.

As was mentioned previously, the pillars in the halls used as gymnasiums presented a challenge to some players. For example, it was common practice to see a defensive player moving backward in an attempt to cover the offensive man strike against one of the pillars. This, of course, created a screen for the offensive man to use to rid himself of the defensive man. This situation helped make players and coaches conscious of the possibilities of using players as screens. Also, as players moved over the court natural screens occurred without previous planning that allowed the offensive man to temporarily be free of the close guarding of the defensive man.

Because of these two factors, an increase in the deliberate use of screens as a part of offensive maneuvers gradually evolved. (By 1930 most good teams used screens when they were stopped from going directly to the basket as their players progressed with the ball from defensive to offensive territory.) Players still played somewhat a territorial position except when a ball was loose or sent out-of-bounds. The forwards often pressed the guards when they attempted to throw the ball downcourt.

Gradually coaches and players conceived of the idea of having the defensive team retreat to the opposite end of the court and wait for the offensive team to advance the ball toward the basket. However, not all of the players came back to protect on defense. The standing forward often remained in offensive territory.

The heavy knee pads worn by most players hindered the speed of movements, but caused players not to hesitate to go into a pile of players in an attempt to secure the ball. However, by the 1915 season the rules were more clearly defined and officiating was made more standard. Thus, play became decidedly less aggressive.

In the early days the standing guard's play was the roughest of all because he was selected for his ability to play aggressively against the opposing high scorer (the standing forward). However, he almost always stood behind the standing forward and attempted to harass him from this position as he shot at the basket. Seldom was there an attempt to intercept the pass made to the forward or to cause the forward to move out of his customary path or position to receive the ball.

The present three-second rule was not in effect so an offensive player could jockey back and forth with the ball as long as he pleased in this area. This rule was not enacted until 1932.

In the very beginning of the game the team defensive and offensive formations used were those adopted from the game of soccer with the forwards receiving the ball in an attempt to score, the centers (left and right) playing in the middle to help intercept the ball or pass to the forwards. The left and right backs, being protectors and passers, were in the back court with the goalie protecting the goal.

Since the basketball court was much smaller in width and length than the soccer field, the territorial division assigned to the various positions was more difficult to define. Most of the players covered most of the court while playing, thereby creating congestion. This factor caused the number of players to be reduced to five.

In the offensive end of the court (when one team had the ball near its own basket), many times only eight players, sometimes nine were stationed there. Four of them would be the defensive players along with four offensive players occasionally augmented by the timid efforts of the standing guard. He was afraid to come too far into the offensive area lest the standing forward (his opponent and the one he was individually responsible for) would receive the ball from a quick long pass and score.

Since the standing forward was expected to shoot often in order to score, he developed a variety of shots which included the hook and fade-away types. Gradually two or more players on the team were able to do in an offensive way what this one player had been doing. The standing forward, as such, gradually faded out of the picture except that he was used on occasions as a stunt by a coach in order to use a sleeper or a "bucket hanger" to confuse the opposing team. However, more probably, the skill of the five offensive players developed to the point that they were able to pass the ball well enough to beat the four defensive players, thus, causing the standing forward, as such, to cease to be functional. When the standing guard could go into offensive territory with confidence that good, sound passing by him and his four teammates could eventually bring about a situation whereby they would find one of their teammates open for a good easy shot, it forced the standing forward to come back on defense. (It is pointed out here that after one of the offensive men scored, the ball was then taken to the center circle for the center jump.) In several games, in the 1922–25 period, the standing forward of both teams waited in vain for a mistake to be made by the five offensive men. Gradually a change took place in the mid-twenties whereby the standing forward began to play on defense.

Early in the history of the game, most of the teams had no or few players of extreme height. Also the center was not a particularly important cog, either offensively or defensively. Gradually, the height and offensive skill of the centers increased until, from a scoring viewpoint, they dominated the game as they do today in many instances. Some few centers were so tall that they could goal tend (intercept the ball in its flight toward the basket) legally since there were no rules in effect concerning this action. Today interference by the defensive player with a ball in its downward flight toward the basket is ruled as a successful shot.

From about 1930 to the present, the pivot/post play of the centers was one of the main means of scoring for many teams. In a sense, the center took the place on offense of the standing forward and on defense the place of the standing guard. In order for the center to keep his prominent place in the high scoring bracket today, he must have help, preferably from high scoring guards who can go around and shoot over the defense. Unless this is true, defensive players converge on the center to the point where it becomes a difficult task for him to receive the ball from his teammates.

The average height of all the players on high school and college teams is increasing. This generally means that a tall center must have something more than height. The top high school, college and professional teams today have outstanding offensive and defensive centers.

The dribble has an interesting history in connection with the early period of the game. It was used at first as a means of escaping from an opponent by the dribbler moving to the rear and it was only through trial and error that it came to be used as an offensive weapon. It was probably by accident that a player eluded his guard and found he could move toward the basket by dribbling the ball. Gradually it was used more and more as an offensive weapon. This was contrary to the way many thought the game should be played, and from 1902 to 1915 a player was not allowed to shoot at the basket after a dribble.

The rule was changed in 1915 to that in use at the present. Then the dribble gradually became more widely used until in the minds of the players and coaches it was being used too much to the detriment of the game. It was even a matter of such great concern in the twenties that the question arose as to whether the dribble should be eliminated entirely from the game.

At various intervals in the past many coaches have prescribed for their players the use that might be made of the dribble. They often have tried to restrict it to a minimum use. Many coaches under this influence considered it poor play to have their players dribble more than two or three bounces before passing or shooting. This attitude was developed because of the "hogging" of the ball by the dribbler when there were players open to whom he could pass the ball.

Gradually a change took place whereby teams even developed team offensive moves and weaves that involved a great amount of dribbling. (In the very early years, such offenses had been used but abandoned.) Fast break moves down the floor were keyed around a dribbler going most of the distance of the court dribbling the ball. Some changes in fast break maneuvers now see many teams pass more than they dribble. However, it does appear that the dribble is here to stay and that every player on a team must know how to use it effectively. Games are won or lost on this ability. Players will enjoy the game more when they have mastered the techniques involved in the proper execution of the dribble.

Shooting the ball at the basket from a position out on the court has changed a great deal during the evolution of the game. In the early days soon after its invention, players tossed the ball toward the basket from a behind-the-head position, or from a chest position in the same manner that the players toss in a soccer ball from out-of-bounds. Some players also tried to shoot the ball much in the same manner as they would throw a baseball. However, this latter type of throw was not particularly successful. Gradually, by trial and error it was discovered that the long under hand throws with two hands were the most successful, especially as the distance from the basket increased. This method of throwing probably developed as players without soccer or rugby experience tried the game. The underhand two-hand motion of shooting is usually tried out first by a young beginner even today.

In the latter portion of the 1915–25 period in the game's development, the top high school and college teams had at least one fine underhand shooter who shot over the defense with uncanny accuracy. In those days many of the defenses retreated to a position near the basket making little or no attempt to press or harass an offensive player out deep on the court. This again stemmed from a soccer concept of team movement. This underhand shooter would then take aim and frequently score. The defenses gradually had to close the distance between the defensive man and the offensive shooter. This caused the offensive shooter to seek other means of scoring (such as two-hand push, fade-away, step-away, and overhead throws). He also learned to fake by his defensive man and to go in toward the basket for close shots. Prior to this stage in the game's development, driving one-hand lay-ups were only used in the game's development, driving one-hand lay-ups were only used when a player was clearly in the open. Actually very early in the game most close shots were taken from a stationary position usually with both feet on the floor.

Using the board as a target for shooting rather than the rim of the basket when attempting medium to long shots was quite common for many years. The players attempted to use the backboard almost exclusively when shooting a long side court shot. This was developed as the underhand style of shooting became prevalent. During the era from about 1914 to 1925 many points were scored by players using the backboard as a target because of the low arc of the ball and the great amount of backward english (spin) the player could put on the ball to cause it to reflect off the backboard into the basket.

As glass backboards began to be used (in the early twenties in some places), it became more difficult to score when striking the backboard because of the decreased friction created between the ball and the glass surface. In addition the partial transparency of the glass offered less of a target than the wooden backboard. Now a rectangular taped outline is often placed on the glass above the basket to aid the shooter in fixing his sight on a target spot, but this aids the close shooter in making setups, etc., more than it does the medium or long shooter. The advent of the fan-shaped backboard (still official) cut down the target surface and opened up wider shooting space, especially at the ends beyond the basket (between the board and the out-of-bounds line).

Finally, the more exclusive use of the one-hand shot from the floor influenced the selection of the shooting target. It is easier to shoot at the rim with the use of the one-hand style because there is less english on the ball and if it strikes the board it is not as apt to go into the basket as is true with the two-hand under-and-overhand (push) shots. It would require more effort on the part of the one-hand shooter to strike the board because of the greater distance and the english necessary to cause the ball to spin firmly backward.

All the reasons mentioned above changed the target area the player used when shooting. This is not to say that the backboard is not now used by some players on shots from the floor. However, the chances of success in shooting for many players has caused a change to take place in reference to the selection of the target.

The individual and team offensive moves we see today largely resulted from what the defensive players or team did and vice versa what the defense did in moving to stop the offensive moves as they developed. However, for the most part it was the defense attempting to catch up to the offense as the game progressed.

In the early days teams played a man-to-man defense. This was a carry-over from the soccer origin. The defensive team retreated under its own basket and waited patiently for the offensive team to move down the court. Since there was no restriction on time nor was the court divided by a middle line, the teams often did not hurry, but moved gradually down the court to their defensive positions. Stalling tactics and use of deliberate styles of play were formulated by the coaches (not players, usually) as devices to upset the opposition. However, for the most part these maneuvers were first seen by the coaches as a result of players accidentally using the moves briefly.

Even the zone defense as it is practiced today and especially in the immediate past was not conceived by the players as a consistent device to use. It may have been used only temporarily or accidentally for a few minutes by players thereby giving some coach the idea of its possibilities. However, the concept of helping out a teammate on defense (as practiced in zone and sagging man-to-man defenses) was not new, even from the beginning since the members of the YMCA class, where the game was invented, were people who had had extensive experience in doing this maneuver when playing soccer and rugby football.

The theory from the origin of the game, then, was that the offensive team came to the defensive team and attempted to score. Nowadays many coaches believe it is the responsibility of the defensive team to force the offensive team to come to the scoring area, especially if the defensive team is behind in the score. However, the present rules are designed to make the offensive team make some attempts offensively.

Individual defensive stance has undergone considerable change during the history of the game. In the early days the guarding player (the player on defense) placed his feet somewhat parallel and apart but hopped about a great deal, while widely flinging his arms in an effort to harass the offensive player when shooting or passing. He could get by with using these tactics because most passes were thrown in the air rather than bounced to the offensive player. Faking by and going toward the basket moves by the offensive player were used infrequently or not at all.

Gradually, as the offensive player began to fake and drive by the defensive man, a defensive stance whereby the body were lowered to enable the guard to move more rapidly to the rear had to be used. Also, the distance away from the offensive man had to be increased. To counter this move made by the defense the offensive player began to shoot over the defense player in the underhand manner mentioned before. This shooting procedure forced the guard to go out after the shooter and the use of a staggered stance with the feet was usually employed to prevent the shooter from driving toward the basket. One arm was raised to prevent the player from shooting and the other arm was lowered to guard against a dribble occurring or a low or bounce pass being made. (The bounce pass was not used very much until after the game was ten or more years old.) This defensive stance mentioned above forced the offensive player to use the two-handed chest shot which was much harder to block because the starting position of the ball was close to the body and the releasing of it was done from a position closer to the height of the head. The two-handed chest shot was at first a cross between the underhand shot and pure two-handed chest shot. It was delivered in a long, low movement of the arms and with a great amount of spin being put on the ball. As the defense player came closer to the offensive player the long sweeping movement made by the arms in shooting gradually were shortened. This caused the ball to go toward the basket in a shorter arc. Shooting on the run with one and two hands was used but still very infrequently. Only occasionally would a player jump into the air and release the ball toward the basket.

The defensive man's play became so good that it was difficult for the shooter to deliver a two-handed chest shot within 20 feet of the basket. The one-hand set shot and various types of jump shots* then became more and more prevalent for use close to the basket. Due to the fact that the one-hand shot is used so much now, many players fail to recognize the advantage of using two hands when shooting the ball from long range. The exclusive use of one-hand shooting means the player usually must be within 20 to 25 feet or closer to the basket in order to have much success in scoring. A good two-handed shooter is able to increase the successful distance 5 to 10 feet and deliver the ball in an easy, unpressed shot.

As soon as the defense became too good for the offense, a special maneuver or a different type of shooting style, usually best adapted to upset the defensive player, became a favorite of top players. This development in turn was seen and copied by others. However, most of the types of shooting styles used today have been used in the past, although usually not as exclusively or successfully by one single individual or team. For example, to say that Hank Luisetti, Stanford University's great forward of yesterday, invented the one-handed shot would be a mistake. Ten years before his time Charles (Chuck) Hyatt, a great player at Pittsburgh University, used a one-handed set shot from the field with great effectiveness, but he had such a variety of shots he never had his one-handed shot popularized as Luisetti did during his playing days. Hyatt, however, did not shoot his one-handed shot on the run and in a jump such as Luisetti often did. Actually the defense was not good enough to make him rely heavily on this one type of shot. Possibly the members of Dr. Naismith's class shot the ball one-handed (in a manner even different from that used in throwing a baseball), but not with the same finesse as displayed today. They undoubtedly did some of this style of shooting because of Naismith's concept that the ball should be tossed at the basket in an arc such as was done in throwing a stone in the duck-on-the-rock game he played as a boy.

Many types of shots and passes were thus used from the very beginning, but as the game became more widely played, if a star player or an entire team consistently used a particular shot successfully, it was soon copied for use by many players in various sections of the country. While a particular style of shooting may have been developed because it was best fitted for use by one specific type of body build and as such might not be advantageous for use by all players, generally speaking, only those styles of shooting that have stood the test of time have lasted until the present day.

*One of the authors is given credit for being the first player to use a jump shot as a primary offensive weapon (see Foreword).

Up to the early thirties the various parts of the country had somewhat their own style of shooting and playing the game. The eastern part of the United States was noted for its two-handed chest style of shooting long set shots. The western part had players who shot more running and jumping types of shots. Today, however, while some of this difference still exists, most players from the East shoot the ball in a similar style to those from the West.

Today, the jump shot is practically the standard shot used from coast to coast. The mobility of the coaching profession and the fact that basketball games are seen on television have tended to eliminate any regional differences in styles of play that might have existed in the past.

Recently, an emphasis on better defense has occurred both in professional, collegiate, and interscholastic basketball play. Scores tend to be lower and defensive skills more highly valued. A similar phenomenon has occurred in both football and baseball. In basketball, part of this recent trend may be attributed to a relaxation of certain rules regarding the degree to which a defensive player may use his hands to maintain contact with his opponent. However, this only partially explains the phenomenon. Often a unified chant of "Defense! Defense!" arises from a crowd. This represents a growing appreciation for defensive skills which can only enhance the overall status of the game.

Soon after the game was invented women began athletic competition in basketball, playing at first under the same rules as men. It is stated that Smith College had competition in basketball in 1892. Four years later, 1896, Stanford University and the University of California (Berkeley) women played intercollegiate basketball.* Competition at the high school level for girls in some regions soon developed and lasted until the end of the 1920's. Rules had been changed earlier for women and girls and women played in many sections of the United States under a "play day" intra-mural atmosphere with a three court division restriction.* Yet in some sections of the country boys and girls in high school teams played basketball under the same rules and conditions after World War I until around 1928. A few states never abandoned highly competitive basketball for girls (notably Iowa).

In the late 1960's women decided to reestablish competition for girls and women on yet a much stronger basis than ever before done in the United States. (Many foreign countries have had strong competition for women for many years.) At the present time, girls and women are playing competitive basketball throughout the nation under similar rules as do the boys and men.

*Rice, E. A.; Hutchinson, J. R.; and Lee, M., *A Brief History of Physical Education,* Ronald Press Co., 1969, p. 197.

Professional basketball is not a new venture. It existed in the east and mid-west from before the 1920's until the late 1940's. The rules under which the game was played were similar to that used in the amateur ranks. One notably exception was that "99 fouls eliminated a player from the game". (This idea has been recently adopted by the American Basketball Association professional league.)

In the early days, trips to games were made in old buses. There was very little money offered as salary and the total number of players participating was small.* Of much greater importance were the AAU teams which were composed of the majority of great college players.

Today the best college players usually join a professional team. The salaries are quite high and the recognition given the players is very great.

Psychology of Coaching Basketball

The importance of psychological factors in coaching winning basketball is known to every coach. Proper recognition and utilization of these factors with a team can often be the difference between a successful and unsuccessful season. Many coaches have proven to be superb motivators of young men. Others have been less than spectacular and have suffered greatly from lack of effort by dissention on a team. Generally, the use of psychological methods with athletes has been developed on a trial and error basis without having any firm foundation in research or theory. Until quite recently this was necessary because the discipline of psychology had little to offer in theory or research that could be translated into practical terms and utilized successfully by a coach. However, there is now a growing interest in what is most commonly referred to as sports psychology. Text books are available in this area and research and theory is growing both in terms of quantity and quality. It is hoped that in the not too distant future a sufficient body of knowledge may exist that will allow proper exposure in this important field during a coach's preservice experience.

The best advice to offer to a coach now is to state that he should progress cautiously and be wary of easy answers to any of his player problems. Human behavior is enormously complex and highly individual. Young men who compete in organized basketball programs are most often initially highly motivated. Their success or failure in basketball may indeed be one of the most important matters in their young lives. This is especially true of certain youngsters during the crucial adolescent years. This places an

*An exception might be the Harlem Globetrotters professional team, and even they had some lean years.

enormous burden on the coach. A situation is created that has the potential for great benefit to the individual, but also for great harm. Many youngsters "find themselves" through their success in basketball. Unfortunately, many others are crushed by their failures in the sport. It is too easy for a coach to remember the former while forgetting the latter.

Perhaps the most important psychological aspect for the coach to recognize is that each player is an individual with a unique genetic and environmental history. Each is born with a different set of abilities and each has been subjected to a different environmental history during the formative years. By the time a youngster reaches the age for participation in formalized age group basketball programs, he already has developed a personality and psychological make-up that is resistant to change. The first task for a coach to perform should be to deal with this human individuality. This is best done by getting to know the youngster as well as possible. This can only be accomplished by knowing how the player behaves off the court as well as during practice. Nothing is more clear than that each individual tends to behave differently in response to different situations. A player may behave in certain ways during basketball practice and differently at home or in a math class or among his peers. By getting to know and recognize that such changeable action exists within the total behavior pattern of a player, a coach can more properly motivate the individual and attempt to cope with any problems that arise during the course of a season.

A coach has the potential to help a player improve not only his basketball performance, but also his general approach to life. However, it must be recognized that sometimes coaches ask players to perform or behave in a manner that is inconsistent with any approach to life that an educational institution should attempt to foster. Even if a basketball coach is concerned solely with performance, his main goal should be to help players overcome their fears and apprehensions and build confidence in themselves concerning their ability to play the game.

There is no doubt that a coach can accomplish his personal goals in basketball through the use of threats, coercion, and punishment. Many coaches are best characterized by such terms, and indeed, it has even become popular to suggest that such kind of treatment is really beneficial to the players' total development as individuals. While there is no doubt that goals can be accomplished in this kind of psychological atmosphere, there is considerable evidence to refute the notion that this is the best way to accomplish goals. Above all, there is no evidence anywhere to suggest that it is psychologically healthy for players to be continually abused with a series of threats, coercions, and punishments. Coaches must scrutinize their beliefs and practices in this area very rigorously to see if they are educationally sound. Too often, coaches attempt to defend practices on the basis of their potential benefit to the player when they are really promoting practices that seem to produce short term performances that benefit the coach. Nothing is more obvious in this situation than to be reminded of the fact that many basketball coaches are extremely successful over a long period of time without having to resort to threats and punishments to motivate their players.

One of the very best methods for a coach to use in motivating players is to help them establish clear set goals. Evidence of progress towards well-defined goals is highly motivating. However, it must be remembered that the goals need to be well defined. A nebulous or ill-defined goal cannot be worked toward, because the individual does not know when progress has been made.

Many learning theorists today agree that there are two basic methods to use to aid humans to learn. One method is through reward. The other is through punishment. Punishment can be an effective tool to use, but it needs to be used wisely and sparingly. Most gains brought about through the use of punishment can be just as easily accomplished by carefully utilizing reward. The strongest rewards in an athletic environment are: (1) the chance to play in games, (2) praise from the coach, and (3) recognition by peers. A pat on the back at the right moment can work wonders with a young basketball player, and, in the long run, the use of positive motivational methods will prove much more satisfying to the coach and the players alike. One crucial step taken is necessary if a coach wants to focus on positive motivational techniques. That step is for the coach to begin to look more for what a player does right than what the player does wrong. Coaches tend to react to mistakes and to errors than they do to good play in performance. A positive motivator tries to focus mainly on those aspects of performance that are accomplished well. This is not to suggest that a coach should not point out and try to correct errors. It only suggests that a better balance between error correction and focus on good performance would produce a much stronger positive environment within which players would be more strongly motivated.

To be good shooters, basketball players must be relaxed, and it is the coach's lot to work toward the attainment of this goal of relaxation for all his players. Players must develop a quiet but sure confidence in their ability to shoot under game pressure. The coach can, no doubt, do his most effective work in this matter in individual consultation with each player. This is particularly true before games. It has recently developed that coaches, players, and spectators alike expect a kind of mad frenzy of emotion from players just before a contest begins. Most of this show of emotions is for the benefit of the fans and has little positive and perhaps undesirable effect on the performance of players. Indeed, a good argument could be raised that it is more likely to prove a real detriment to performance than it is an aid in performance to some players. In fact, some players probably play better when they react to a pep talk given by the coach. These players need to be "fired up." However, other players probably perform better when the coach calms them down by saying very little before a game. This tends to negate the idea of a team pep talk, at least one that is designed to create a high level of emotional tension.

Regardless, it is unlikely that a coach will be able to get his team up for each game on the schedule. This is especially true in basketball where a large number of games is to be played. For a coach whose team has a losing record, the problem of getting the players prepared psychologically to play well becomes a constant problem. This is particularly true for his players in games where the team is likely to be well outmanned. For a winning coach, the problems are quite different. A winning coach has to examine his schedule carefully to pinpoint the games he believes the team should be best prepared for psychologically. If he tries to get his team "up" for every game, he will be unable to get that little extra from his team in a particularly crucial game.

Another factor that must be considered in the psychology of coaching basketball is now mentioned. Recently, a great flurry of research has been done attempting to relate personality traits to performance in various sports. It is no longer uncommon for players to take psychological tests (such as the Cattel 16 P.F.) and for the outcome of these tests to be used by coaches in selecting, evaluating, and placing his players. A strong note of caution must be raised on this point. This type of research is in its infancy and has been scrutinized and often highly criticized within the discipline of sports psychology. Until the research instruments in this field become a great deal more sophisticated than they are now, it would be wise for the coach to use such information sparingly, and never to yield to the temptation to place test result information above his own personal observations of the player's behavior. Indeed, the coach should take a generally skeptical attitude towards information generated from paper and pencil tests. Any advice generating from results received from paper and pencil data is highly inferential, and should be used with caution. This is not to suggest that such information has no value. Rather, the information should be interpreted carefully and considered in light of the coach's total knowledge of the player.

There are many other issues that could be dealt with under the topic of psychology of coaching basketball. Indeed, textbooks on the psychology of coaching are now appearing on the market. It is probably sufficient at this point to state that the good coach will recognize that there are certain aspects of his job that are truly psychological in nature and that he will have to deal with them accordingly. For example, the coach must recognize that his handling of the players on the bench is a crucial factor in the success of his team. Likewise, the treatment of players during practices can produce strong positive or negative psychological benefits for a team. We think it is legitimate for a coach to consider the general behavior of players when selecting a team, and, if necessary, to eliminate a player solely because of the potential psychological damage that might accrue to the team by his presence.

Many other factors can also psychologically affect a player, and thus are legitimate concerns for the coach. Some of these are reflected in the series of questions that follows. What does each player do during the afternoon before a home game? How does the pre-game meal affect a player psychologically? Who is permitted to accompany the team on an away trip? What superstitions do the players have? Does a particular superstition help or hinder the performance of a given player? These are some questions that a coach will have to consider when looking for the psychological cue that will help his team to achieve a high level game performance and his players to find satisfaction in playing the game as well as they can under the circumstances.

Principles of Motor Learning as Applied to the Learning of Basketball Skills

A great deal of research in the area of learning has been conducted by many investigators in many disciplines. Since World War II, a special area of investigation has been identified as "motor learning," which refers specifically to the learning of physical skills. Much of the research has been haphazard and unsophisticated, as might be expected in a relatively young science. However, there is now a sufficient body of research literature available to begin to identify valid principles of learning for sport skill situations and to do so on the basis of scientific evidence rather than pedagogical (coaching) opinion. Many coaches have effectively applied learning principles for years without being aware that they had any basis in research or theory. Over the years the methods that "work" tend to be similar to those that might be developed from theory. Nonetheless, it is important that potential young coaches develop sound coaching methods during their training rather than having to depend on years of trial and error.

There are many factors that affect the rate at which a basketball player learns the skills of the game. Not all of these factors can be controlled by a coach. In this section an attempt is made to propose a select set of principles that the coach or teacher may follow in coaching and teaching situations.

Learning principles proposed for use in basketball learning situations are:

1. Motivation is probably the single most important factor affecting the rate at which players acquire skill and perform well.
2. Positive motivational techniques have greater long term payoffs than do negative motivational techniques.
3. Feedback is a necessary condition for effective learning.
4. Artificial feedback can be effectively used to create a better learning situation.
5. Clear goals are important to effective learning.
6. Practice must be active and purposeful for all participants in order to be effective.
7. Players learn to perform well under the stress of game conditions when some stress is introduced into practice sessions.
8. The length of the practice session, if well planned and not beyond reason, should not affect the amount of learning.
9. Mental practice can improve learning and performance.
10. Skills and strategies should be learned as meaningful wholes.
11. Skills should be learned somewhere near the speed at which they will be performed.
12. Verbalization by the coach is of limited usefulness and should seldom replace active participation.
13. Modeling is a powerful learning method and should be utilized frequently.
14. Practices will be most conducive to learning when clear goals and consequences are stated and utilized.

It is an embarrassing but a true axiom that a motivated learner will learn and perform despite the teacher and teaching method used. Certainly, every coach is aware of cases where diligent youngsters have become very skilled basketball players by practicing on their own at a backyard hoop and later perfecting their skills in a local church or YMCA league. Motivation is probably the single most important ingredient in learning and performance, and coaches would do well to focus their attention on this important variable. It should be noted that a distinction has been made between learning and performance. This is a distinction that is too often overlooked. Learning means acquiring a skill not currently within the skill repertoire of an individual or team. Learning situations require certain factors to be present for efficient acquisition of new skills. Performance means the degree to which an acquired skill is performed in any given situation or at any given time. Obviously, while coaches are extremely interested in learning, the more important and difficult task is to develop an approach to coaching that maximizes the performance of the players. Seldom are games lost because players have not learned sufficient skills to win. However, games are often lost because players do not perform at a level commensurate with their level of skill development. Much of what is discussed in this section pertains specifically to creating an efficient learning situation. Many factors potentially affect the learning situation. However, it can be stated unequivocally that motivation is the factor of paramount importance in performance.

Coaches can motivate performance through the use of positive or negative techniques. Although both work, a strong case can be made for the long term benefits of utilizing a positive motivational approach to coaching. This is true not only for performance, but also for the many important side effects that accrue from the positive motivational approach. It should be stated clearly that positive motivational techniques do not necessarily imply fostering a boisterous, rah-rah approach to coaching. While a great deal of enthusiasm can work wonders with individuals and teams, coaches must be careful that their positive approaches are genuine and appropriate to the individuals with whom they are working in a day-to-day setting.

Negative motivational techniques may produce short term benefits, but often create problems in the longer run. It is a basic law of human behavior that we tend to approach situations that have positive consequences and avoid situations that regularly produce negative consequences. Coaches who rely heavily on punishment, coercion, negative discipline, and a generally hardline approach will eventually find that they have youngsters who will not stay out for the team unless they know they are going to play. They also will often have discipline and dissention problems. Most importantly, they will have failed in their educational function because they will have lost the opportunity to favorably influence the player.

Feedback is information that results from a response. It is most often used to make slight changes in the next response. For example, a player uses the feedback from a missed shot to make a slight change in his delivery technique. Over a period of years, with the enormous number of trials that a player has in skills such as in shooting and passing, a behavior pattern emerges. Feedback is absolutely necessary to learning. Fortunately, there is ample feedback that is intrinsic to playing basketball. The player knows when he missed a shot, made a bad pass, or got faked out of position.

The comments a coach makes to a player about his skills are labeled artificial feedback, in the sense that they are not intrinsic to playing basketball. Often the intrinsic feedback gives one message, but it may not always be the message the coach wants to convey. For example, a player makes a cross-court pass that is successful, but the coach must point out to him that such passes have high probabilities of being intercepted. If the pass is intercepted, the message is clear.

Coaches can also create artificial feedback devices that provide extra information, and do not require the coach's constant presence. Generally speaking, the more precise the feedback, the quicker is the skill development. Artificial feedback can often add extra information to the intrinsic feedback. For example, many coaches want their players to jump straight up when shooting a jump shot off the dribble. Players have a tendency to let their bodies carry forward in the direction of their movement. Often, simply putting down on the floor some tape markers can help players to overcome their tendency to stray on the moving jump shot. The tape markings could be graded in 3-inch distances. Players could dribble quickly to the shot mark, shoot the jump shot, and then look down to see how far from the jump mark they landed. This artificial feedback (the tape on the floor) will help them to improve their skill at jumping straight up without having to have the coach present to verbally inform them about the amount of stray that takes place in their jump shots.

The example just discussed leads to another important point. Players in order to learn skill efficiently, must have clear goals. It is not sufficient to simply tell players that they should jump straight up on their jump shot and then leave them to practice without having any specific goal or specific feedback. Quicker and more lasting improvement will occur when players know that they must shoot 40 jump shots a day from a fast dribble and land within 6 inches of their landing jump mark. Clearly specified practice goals are crucial. Players should never just run laps. The inevitable result of simply running laps is that the coach has to chide and reprimand the players to get them to run hard. This latter action violates the positive motivation principle. It would be far better for both the player and coach if clear performance goals were set up for each practice. Fifty laps done in a certain amount of time makes clear to the individual player what must be accomplished. Likewise, twenty five sprints, each run under a certain time criterion, makes it unnecessary for the coach to stand and yell at players who tend to loaf. When a player runs a sprint that is above the allotted time, it simply does not count as a sprint and must be done over. The precision and clarity of the performance goal helps the player and coach to know how much improvement is being made and diminishes the necessity for the coach to act as a disciplinarian and traffic director.

Practice must be active and purposeful for the player in order for learning to take place. The more the player participates, the better are the chances for learning. This concept must be kept in mind when the coach plans drills, scrimmages, and chalk-talks. The time spent in practice must not only be active, but also purposeful. Practice will result in no improvement, no matter how much time is spent at it unless it is purposeful. The classic example of this may be found in handwriting which is practiced a great deal but seldom results in any improvement. The same may be said for most "free shooting" done at the start of practice. Unless shooting is purposeful, no improvement will occur. The 15 or 20 minutes allotted to shooting prior to the beginning of organized practice can be very meaningful if clear goals are established and feedback is monitored by the coach or a manager.

A practice session that is conducted in a completely relaxed atmosphere is probably not best suited to learning. Basketball skills must be performed under pressure. While it is the goal of every coach to help his players learn to perform in a confident, relaxed manner, this will seldom be accomplished in a completely relaxed practice environment. Confident, relaxed performance is the result of learning how to perform skills in a pressure situation, so that the pressure is diminished or ignored. This will occur only when there is some pressure in practice, so that players can learn to adapt to it. The pressure atmosphere of game competition must be approximated in the practice environment. While it is never possible to totally or accurately recreate game pressure, it nonetheless is a useful goal to attempt to create some pressure and then help the players to find ways to perform well despite the pressure.

The length of a practice session should not deter from the learning potential. It was long felt that players could not learn while mentally or physically fatigued. However, all research findings seem to indicate that while performance may lessen toward the end of a long practice session, players are still fully capable of learning new skills or strategies. However, the coach should be aware that performance may drop off under such circumstances, but, this should not unduly excite him. New offensive and defensive maneuvers can still be learned even though players may look a bit ragged as they perform the newly learned patterns. Changing activities within practice sessions is probably the best way to keep players as mentally and physically alert as possible.

Mental practice is the act of thinking about a skill, strategy or game experience. Naturally, mental practice can occur in between practice sessions. There is abundant evidence to support the notion that mental practice can improve skill. This is particularly true if some effort is made by the coach to direct the nature of that mental practice and also to have it be a positive mental experience. There is also evidence to suggest that pregame mental rehearsal in which the player imagines himself as being successful is helpful to game performance. However, there is no evidence anywhere to suggest that mental practice is better than actual physical practice.

Generally speaking, learning with the use of the whole method is superior to learning by the part method. A whole should be defined as a meaningful unit, and the size of the unit is best determined by the developmental level of the player. The jump shot, for instance, is best taught by the whole method right from the outset, no matter what level of performance the player has attained. Players possessing higher levels of skill can practice parts of a skill to great advantage, but they know the skill well enough so that they fill in the rest of the movements of the skill mentally and therefore are really practicing a meaningful whole. The question of the use of part and whole methods of learning becomes very crucial when teaching an offense to a team. The coach should make sure that if the offense is too intricate to learn as a whole, the parts selected for learning should be as large as the learners can comprehend without getting unnecessarily confused with trying to understand the whole.

Skills should be learned at somewhere near the speed at which they will have to be performed. Forsaking speed for the cause of accuracy is not good procedure. A combination of emphases being placed on speed and accuracy is no doubt the best method to use, but when a question arises as to a choice between the two, it is best to utilize a speed emphasis in practice rather than an accuracy emphasis. Practice on accuracy in the skill of passing, for example, usually will not transfer when the skill has to be used at game speed.

Verbalization by the coach is a greatly overused method of teaching, especially as it applies to the beginning learner. The player will have to have rather full command of a skill vocabulary before verbalization will have much meaning to him, and a young player seldom has sufficient command of the skill vocabulary to respond properly to this method. At any learning level the use of verbalization by the coach should not replace practice time that could be more meaningfully spent in active participation by the player. A basketball player learns and improves most by doing the skill and not as much by listening to someone else tell him about the skill. Perhaps a short time spent in the classroom before practice where discussion of the skills desired is conducted might be very valuable to clarify certain points so that maximum active participation may take place once actual practice begins on the floor. On the other hand, verbalization by a player is extremely important so that the greatest possible understanding may result.

Demonstration still remains as the single best method of teaching skills, and coaches who no longer can demonstrate skills well should rely upon assistants or on their more highly skilled players to perform this function. "One picture is truly worth a thousand words" if that picture is a live demonstration done by a skilled player. The use of the videotape recorder provides for the live demonstration to be presented in slow motion. Also the errors made by a player may be viewed by him with the use of such a device.

It may well be that use of videotape replays will revolutionize motor skills teaching in the future. There is good reason to believe that expert demonstration of a skill combined with videotape replay of the learner's efforts might afford an optimum learning environment. The amount of feedback information that the learner gets from viewing his efforts on videotape far exceeds the amount of feedback information that can be gained by any other known method. The learner can, in effect, compare his performance with that of the expert. This method of teaching motor skills could greatly reduce the amount of time generally thought necessary to spend for the perfection of complex sports skills.

Skills and strategies can be learned by watching someone else perform them. Obviously, this is well known and the use of demonstration is evidence of its widespread use. However, the general method of watching someone else perform can be used in other ways. The psychological term used to describe this phenomenon is "modeling." Several factors affect the success of modeling. The most important is the success or failure of the model. Do not expect players to attempt to learn techniques or strategies that appear to be unsuccessful. Another factor is the degree to which the individual player relates to the model. This is why so many youngsters try to imitate a Walt Frazier or a Pete Maravich. Often this modeling effect is beneficial, but sometimes it can prove detrimental to the performance of the player. Coaches can use modeling at almost any point in practice. Whenever a good play has been made, the coach can stop practice and call attention to the play and the player who performed it. The rest of the players will quickly get the message. It must be remembered, however, that the success of the model is crucial. If a coach praises a great effort by a player in practice but that player does not get more chance to play in games, then eventually the rest of the players will learn that the coach's praise in practice really does not pay off; thus, the modeling effect will be greatly diminished.

In summary, practices will be most conducive to learning when clear goals are established and consequences are stated and utilized. When players learn that a lap run above a criterion time does not count as a lap, they will quickly put forth the effort necessary to meet the criterion time. This means that the coach must plan carefully for each practice. He must spend more time attempting to manage his practice sessions properly and monitor the performance of his players during practice so effectively as to provide feedback and utilize consequences. Student managers can be of great help in performing some of these tasks for the coach.

How to Understand and Enjoy Watching a Basketball Game

Often times the high school coach (also the college coach) is asked to make a talk at the school assembly, downtown service club, girls' league, mothers' club, or to any group representing the school or the community. One of the topics that he might select is that of "How to Understand and Enjoy Watching a Basketball Game." In addition, the same information could be presented to the physical education classes for discussion by and for the students' better enjoyment of the season's varsity games.

Some of the ideas that might help promote better understanding and enjoyment of the game are as follows:

1. Identification of the colors worn by each team is made. This should include the shoes if they are different so that the spectator knows at once which team has possession of the ball, etc.

2. A brief review is given of the following rules, such as:

a. The ten-second rule means than an offensive team has only ten seconds to bring the ball past the center line of the court after securing possession in some way from the other team in the back court. Failure to do so results in loss of the ball.

b. An offensive player cannot remain in the lower half of the key, from the foul line or on to the end line, longer than three seconds with or without the ball. Penalty is loss of the ball. However, any offensive player can remain as long as he chooses in the outer half of the key. The defensive players may play any place on the floor they choose without penalty. The three second lane rule coverage applies only when the ball is located in the offensive half of the court.

c. Personal fouls are those fouls committed by a player which involve body contact with an opponent while the ball is in play or is being thrown in from out-of-bounds. A common foul is a personal foul which is neither flagrant nor intentional nor committed against a player trying for a field goal. A player is awarded a free throw for a common foul committed by a player of the opposing team beginning with that team's seventh personal foul in a half of a game played in halves, or fifth personal foul in a half of a game played in quarters. At this point a bonus free throw is awarded for each common foul, provided the first free throw is successful.

d. Technical fouls are those fouls committed by a player that do not involve contact or any unsportsmanlike action while the ball is dead. Use of abusive language is included in this category.

e. Any player who commits 5 personal fouls (6 in professional games) must leave the game and cannot return even if the teams are tied in score at the end of the regulation time and play an overtime period.

f. Any other rules (including new ones) of any consequence including those on foul shooting, goal tending, common fouls, bonus shots, and restraining lanes or areas should be made known.

3. The home team's basket is known. This can be found out as soon as the two teams line up for the first center jump. The centers must face

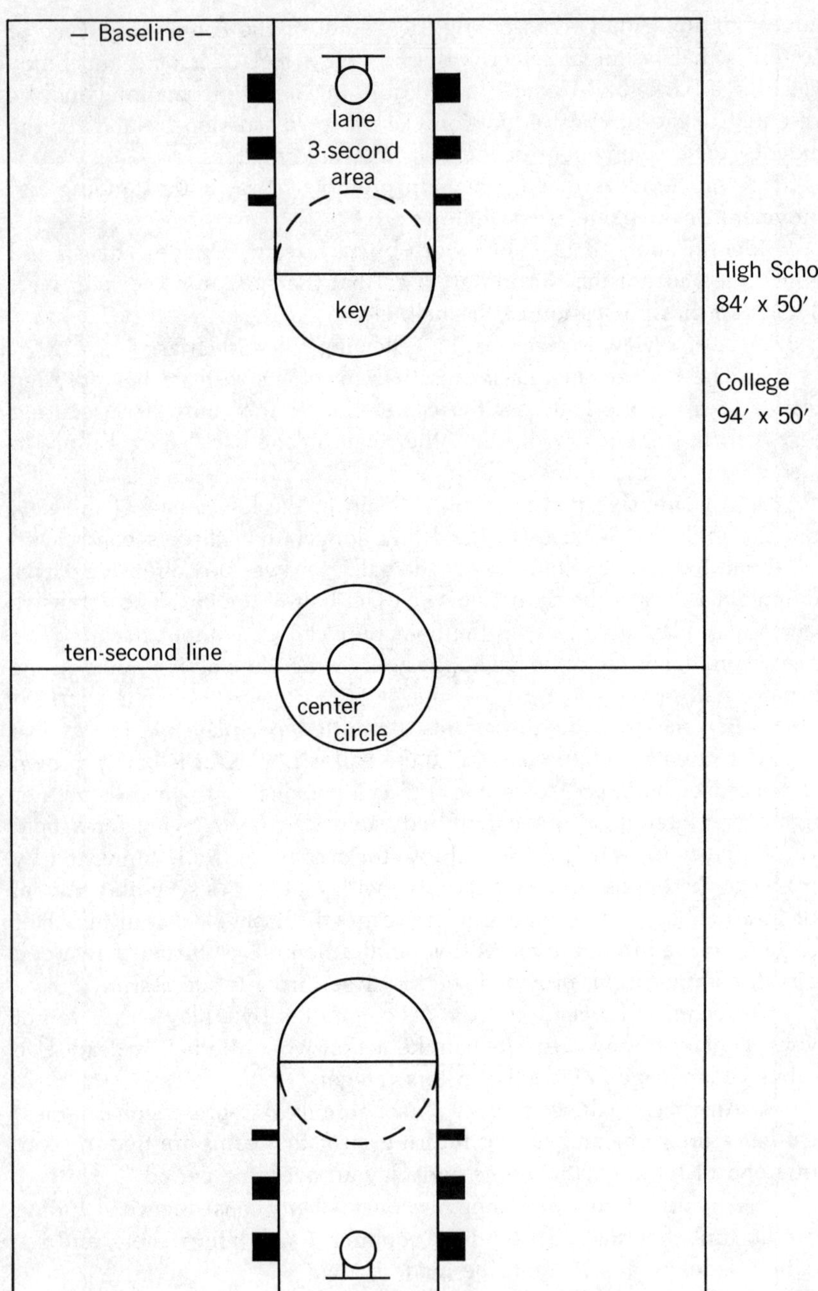

Diagram of a basketball court.

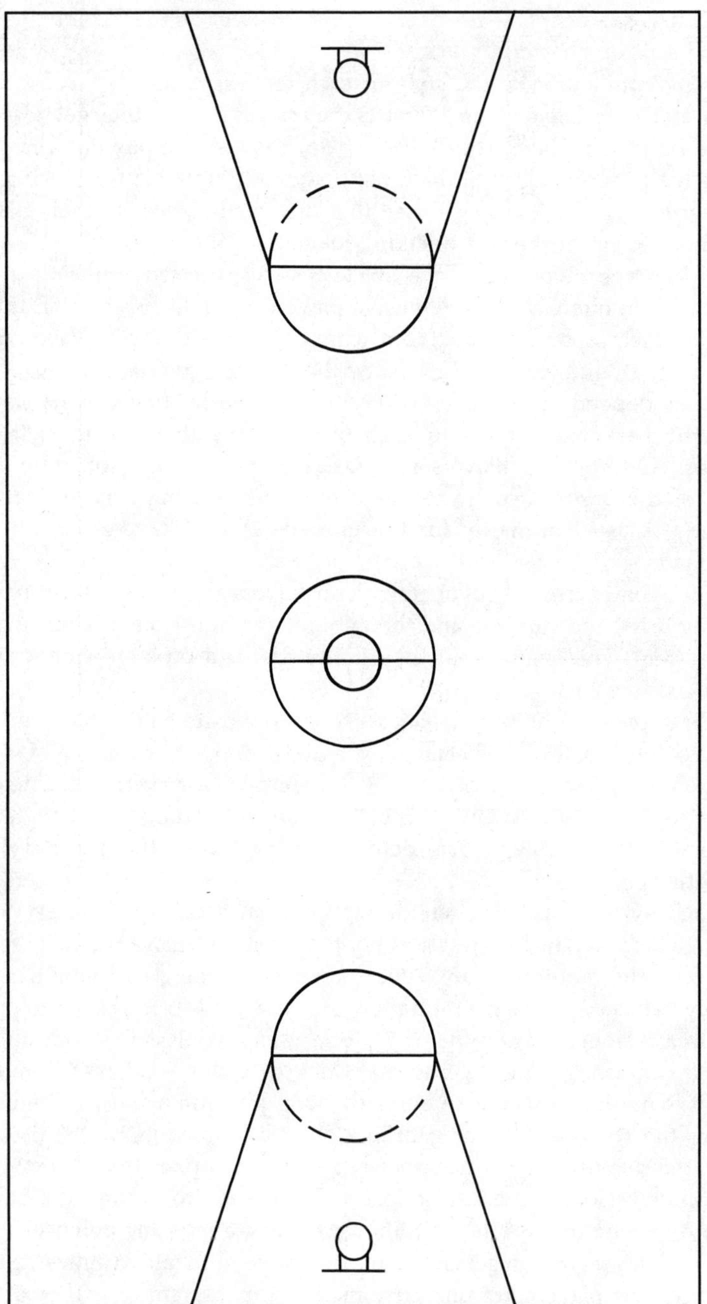

Diagram of a future basketball court.

their own baskets. The teams exchange baskets at the beginning of the second half or quarter.

4. Determination of the style of each team is made.

a. Do both teams run as fast as they can as soon as they get possession of the ball in the back court? If they do, they are employing a *fast break.* If one team fast breaks, but the other one does not, the latter is using a *slow break* or *deliberate style of play.* Often this latter team slows up their attack all the more to upset the fast breaking team.

b. After the players of the two teams cross the center line, the manner in which the offensive and defensive players place themselves on the floor signifies their system of play. If one team on offense puts one player, usually a tall one, around close to the basket, they are using a *single low post* system and they depend on this player to score frequently. Two players stationed near the basket and close to each other means they are using a *double low post.* One or two players stationed out beyond the foul line and in front of the basket usually means a *high post* is being used. Usually this player(s) is used primarily for the purpose of feeding the ball off to his teammates.

If the center area is kept open with no players around this territory except as they drive and run into and then go out again, the team is using an *open lane* system. This means that they do not depend on a tall center as their main scoring threat.

On defense if the players retreat to the opposite end of the court when they lose the ball and if each player plays opposite a player of the opposition they are using a *man-to-man* defense. However, if the team retreats to a spot and follows the ball within the confines of their territory or zone, they are using a *zone* defense. In the future, this latter style may be outlawed.

Each system has its strengths and weaknesses. It is hardest to pass through a zone, but easiest to shoot over it. A man-to-man defense is generally the more popular system and a team using it maintains a more evenly balanced defensive formation. However, it is often easier to pass the ball to a teammate when the opposition uses it (unless the opposing team uses a contesting type defense, in which case this weakness is reduced), but, it is harder to secure an open shooting position against it. Its use also makes the responsibility of guarding one man much more definite.

If the defensive team does not retreat to the opposite end of the court when possession of the ball is lost and proceeds to harrass the offensive team by trying to steal the ball, they are using a pressing defense. The use of this defense will upset many teams and is difficult to move against if the offensive players are unaccustomed to this system or if they are poor dribblers or ball handlers.

5. The best players are identified by name on each team. The recent newspaper accounts may contain this information.

6. The size and ability of players as they warm up prior to the game is observed. Size is only one criterion for success; ability or skill is much more important.

7. As the game continues a note is made as to what player on each team seems to direct the play, especially on offense. He is often called a quarterback.

8. Generally one team uses one style of shooting over another—more hook shots, one-hand, or jump shots are taken. Identification of all shooting styles should be learned.

9. The two coaches are observed to see how they are reacting to stresses occurring during the game. Are they able to keep calm and cool? Some of them have some very amusing antics that they use.

10. A glance occasionally made at the crowd during a tense moment is revealing. It will help the spectator to simmer down and be more rational.

11. The spectator should not always follow the ball, but he should observe the players who do not have the ball. Some of the most unusual happenings have occurred to players and spectators away from where the ball is located at a given moment.

12. Some of the sports language used by the players in describing their own moves and plays should be understood.

13. The officials are a part of the game and should be given some notice, but it should be remembered that their sole duty is to see that the game is conducted properly and orderly. They should not overshadow or rival the players for attention from the spectators. Watching the officials try to decide honestly on making correct decisions may calm down the spectators' booings when decisions go contrary to their wishes.

14. Practice sessions should be visited, if such is permitted, to learn how the home team is progressing and to become more familiar with the players and their habits.

15. Each player has particular moves he likes best to make and he has certain weaknesses and strengths in ability. It is interesting to have first hand knowledge of such information. For example, many players prefer to dribble with the dominant hand when under pressure from the defense.

16. It is well to remember that basketball is a game involving the element of chance. On a given night the weakest team in the league may defeat the best. Thus spectators should keep on cheering for their team.

17. Appreciation for good play and clever moves made by players on either team is shown by giving recognition where it is due.

18. Interest in the game may be heightened by keeping records of the team's accomplishments and miscues made during a game.

Predictions for the Future

An individual who has the spell of the soothsayers upon him feels no compunction when it comes to prophesying how the game of basketball will be played in the future. Thus he sets about doing this task with no thought that he could be wrong in his forecast. However, the following predictions have been made by attempts to combine a measure of common sense, a look at some obvious contemporary trends, and a bit of pure conjecture. There are also certain historical trends that can serve as guides upon which predictions can be made. Some of the guiding principles upon which the foretelling was done are as follows:

1. Infrequent and accidental successful use of certain moves and skills have sometimes provoked their general adoption.
2. Constant study and exchange of views between coaches and players provides a consistent framework for change.
3. New ideas are often borrowed from other games.
4. Periodic review of the game's history reveals that new ways of utilizing old methods and skills that have been popular in the past has been done.
5. Unusual physical builds and/or exceptional talents of players sometimes introduces a new way to perform a skill.
6. The accent on speed of movement in playing the game has consistently increased throughout the years causing new approaches to the game to be introduced.
7. The public has consistently favored the offensive phases of the game thereby creating a favorable attitude toward new developments in this area.
8. Players usually accent the offensive portions of the game in their unsupervised practices. In fact, unusual and new ways of scoring have been developed by the players in these informal sessions.
9. Many new unexpected changes came about even though new rules were adopted for different purposes.
10. Participants in the game have become taller, larger, faster, and more skilled each year.
11. Changes in the rules including restrictions on time spent in certain playing areas continues to increase.
12. New ideas concerning the design of the ball, board, goal, and uniforms continue to be developed.
13. Changes in emphasis such as the coaches stressing defense and the spectators enjoying it, cause acceptance of certain new concepts.
14. International play will introduce new approaches to the playing of the game.

A prediction of things to come shall now be attempted, keeping in mind the above general statements. How soon these predicted ideas will materialize, or indeed, whether they ever will, or not, is up to the basketball personnel of today and of tomorrow. The ideas presented here are not necessarily presented in the order in which it is thought they might become actually part of the game. Rather they are listed as they were conceived without any reference being made to a chronological arrangement.

1. Rules will be explored to determine what possibilities for use of new legal moves exist within the confines of the present language. For example, it is legally possible under the present rules for a foul shooter to dribble or run up to the foul line, jump into the air toward the basket, and release the ball before returning to the floor. Many teams now have a player who on attempting to throw the ball in from out of bounds under the basket may run up and down the base line to elude defensive pressure. These are examples of possibilities for the use of new strategy that is legal within the interpretation of the present rules.

2. Greater knowledge of the time it takes to do various phases of the game in relation to the distance to be traveled by a player and the ball will be known. Also better knowledge is needed as to when the clock is running and when time is out during a game. Concerning the former, the time it takes to dribble the length of the floor, the time it takes to throw the ball in from out of bounds, and the time it takes to move the ball the length of the floor with various types of passes will be more fully explored. Present day players often do not have sufficient knowledge of these aspects of the game to employ complete strategy in relation to their use.

3. Increased emphasis will be placed on the passing game. Ability to pass quickly with speed and on the run will be further developed. Teams will possess more than one or two good passers. Passing will be more fully utilized to keep the defense off balance.

4. Players will increasingly develop the ability to shoot and score on the run. Only occasionally are the current crop of top players able to shoot effectively while moving at great speed.

5. Players will increasingly develop the ability to shoot very quickly after receiving a pass or picking the ball up from the dribble. Preparation for executing the shot will be made before receiving the pass and/or while dribbling.

6. Increased attention will be paid to the weaknesses and limitations of human movement. Players will utilize this knowledge in many ways, especially in attempts to stop the star player.

7. Habits of players will be more closely observed, such as the locations on the floor from which they like to shoot. The defense will then take advantage of the possession of this knowledge.

8. There will be a continued trend toward the complete elimination of specialists. The demand will increasingly be for multi-skilled players. Players

will be able to play either the inside or outside positions on the court and the distinctions between traditional positions will become blurred. The possible exception may be the unusually tall center.

9. New shots will continue to be developed, and they will become increasingly difficult to master and execute. Universal adoption of the three-point rule will increase the value of the long shot. This will also bring about the return of the two-hand set shot as a long distance weapon. The "jump-hook" will be used increasingly by almost all players while they have their backs to the basket. The distance from the basket for its effective use will be increased.

10. International rules will become official. The ten-second rule will be eliminated, the Olympic lane will be adopted, and a shooting time limit—probably a thirty-second rule—will be adopted at all levels of basketball.

11. The change in rules, especially the elimination of the ten-second rule, will allow teams to use the entire floor for offensive and defensive maneuvers in a more complete way.

12. The "fouling-out" rule will be eliminated in favor of more stringent penalties for players who foul frequently. A time penalty may be adopted, such as is used in hockey. The problem of fouling will continue to be the major source of trouble in terms of criticism of the game from the public and also from the coaches' viewpoint. The American Basketball Association (professional) has experimented with the "no foul out" rule. It has been reported that even though the opposing team shoots free throws when a player picks up his seventh and all fouls thereafter (the player may remain in the game) and also gains possession of the ball out-of-bounds, the impact has been rather subtle without essentially changing the game.

13. There will be a lengthening of the distance from the basket to the out-of-bounds line, up to maybe 10 or more feet. This will increase interest in the game by providing the opportunity for the development of new techniques. Out-of-bound plays will have to be changed in order to be utilized in the new area. Also, fewer balls will go out-of-bounds with the additional area providing greater space in which to retrieve it. This change will also help eliminate one source of danger to the players by adding the extra distance for them to stop after shooting a lay-up.

14. Officiating will be less technical but more accurate. One official will be suspended on a track high above the court on a set of wires with mechanical devices that will enable him to move directly over the players in order to observe infractions of the rules. He will use a microphone to communicate his decisions to the players and other officials on the court.

15. Taller players will increasingly take over the function of the "little" man, but there may be an over-all leveling off of the emphasis on pure height alone. The players from 6 feet 4 inches to 6 feet 8 inches will dominate

some aspects of play as they combine the quickness of the smaller man and the jumping ability to match the height of the bigger man.

16. Team strategy will increasingly be determined by the game situation. Teams will use their five best shooters under certain conditions, and their five best defensive players on certain occasions. For overall strategy coaches will increasingly choose their five best players regardless of height. A place on the team will be found for them and team strategy will be accordingly planned.

17. Zone defenses as such will be eliminated due to rule changes and restrictions will continue to be placed on the extremely tall man, such as the recent "no dunking" rule (high school and college) has done. There will be much discussion about raising the height of the goals, but other measures, such as the three-point scoring rule, are more likely to be adopted first.

18. Individual offense and defense play will become more mobile. Aggressive play will increase, especially on defense. Team offensive and defensive plans will be developed with careful consideration being given to the increased mobility and quickness of the players.

19. Three officials in a game will become universal.

The above suggestions certainly do not exhaust the possibilities that could be presented about the predicted changes that may occur in the game of basketball. They stand merely as prognostications made by two extremely interested basketball observers. It appears from what is now known that these are ones that seem most likely to occur in the immediate future. Increased international participation in basketball will tend to standardize the rules used throughout the world. This in turn will help increase world spectator interest in the game. Also, this situation may bring about unforeseen new developments in play.

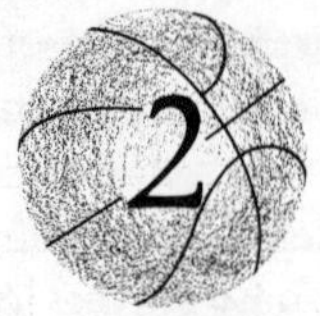

*Individual Player Fundamentals**

Introduction to Principles of Performance in Individual Offensive and Defensive Skills

This chapter contains principles of performance pertaining to individual offensive and defensive skills. An attempt has been made to exclude those techniques, or variations of techniques, that are primarily outcomes of a particular coaching philosophy or have been developed as the result of planned team strategy. What remains, it is hoped, are those underlying principles of performance that must be considered essential or fundamental to successful performance in selected basketball skills, regardless of the coaching philosophy or the team strategy involved. It should be recognized that there are many theories and opinions concerning what are the essential fundamentals of basketball, but no attempt is made here to present all conflicting opinions. Rather, an attempt is made to select those essential techniques of performance which it is believed are the best ones. However, where there are legitimate reasons for having conflicting viewpoints, both or several viewpoints are presented.

It is a moot point as to what is the rank or order of importance of the various categories of fundamentals. The viewpoint which is held about this question will be predicated almost entirely on one's total outlook toward

*In a discussion with Beatrice Gorton, coach of the women's basketball team, Indiana University, Bloomington, she suggested that skill is skill and is not to be regarded as different in relation to sex. Taking into consideration some small physical differences, previous sociological and training experiences, we believe women can play as well as men. So it is believed, that the objective of basketball play, philosophically, should be to harvest the best in play so that continuous comparison will not be made between men and women but that excellence of performance will be noted and valued regardless of the sex of the performer.

the game, and indeed, can serve as the best indication of one's philosophy of basketball. The order in which the various fundamental skills should be learned is more of a legitimate area of debate, and one in which opinion may have been subordinated to that of sound logical thinking. Of all the various skills that can be considered fundamental to basketball, dribbling is most likely the first skill that should be learned. This is true because offensive skills are more difficult to learn than defensive skills and take a great deal longer to perfect, and it also is true because the vast majority of offensive skills are predicated upon the use of the dribble. Passing and receiving should probably be learned next, and are probably best learned together. Shooting should be learned next, and thus the order of dribbling, passing, and shooting is established. It is a matter of fact that offensive basketball is based upon the player being able to dribble, pass, and receive before he shoots at the basket. Thus, it seems quite natural and logical that the three (or four) main offensive skills be learned in that order.

Dribbling

Dribbling refers to the usually oft repeated, one-handed bouncing of the ball against the floor done by an offensive player. It is one of the many fundamental basketball skills that a player must master. Dribbling is considered by many not to be the most important offensive skill, but it should, perhaps, be the first skill that the young player learns to do. If a player is unable to dribble adequately, he will not be able to be as effective as he could be offensively. Thus, dribbling is significant in its direct contribution to offensive play. Therefore, disregarding the small number of real giants (they may be able to play effectively with a minimum of dribbling skill) now present in basketball, it may be stated fairly that dribbling is absolutely essential to effective offensive play. To illustrate its importance, the dribble is employed in advancing the ball into the offensive court, in executing offensive maneuvers, in driving to the basket, in stalling, in fast breaking, and in almost all offensive situations that a player might encounter during a game.

Many coaches are prone to speak disparagingly about the development of the skill of dribbling. This is unfortunate because it tends to convey the impression that dribbling should be often avoided and used only when there is no alternative left by which to advance the ball. Misuse of any skill should be discouraged, but the misuse of a skill does not alter the great importance of that skill to the game of basketball. One does not have to watch a basketball game at any level for any length of time in order to become aware of the significant role that dribbling plays in offensive basketball.

PRINCIPLES OF PERFORMANCE

1. Dribbling at a high level of performance is a kinesthetic and tactile skill, not a visual skill.

2. The height that the ball is dribbled is determined by the proximity of the defensive player and the offensive need at the moment.

3. The dribbler should hold his head up when dribbling the ball so that he may see the other players on the floor.

4. The dribbler should have the confidence and ability to dribble with either hand equally effectively.

5. The ball in dribbling is controlled with the use of the inside portion of the fingertips.

6. The low dribble is accomplished by finger flexion-extension and some wrist flexion-extension.

7. The faster and higher the ball is dribbled the more wrist flexion-extension (and even to some extent elbow flexion-extension) is utilized.

8. The low, controlled dribble is executed with the knees flexed, the hips lowered, and the trunk kept straight.

9. The fast dribble is executed by having less flexion in the knees and raising the hips as the center of mass of the dribbler goes forward and upward.

10. The faster the dribble is executed the more the ball is pushed out in front of the dribbler. The dribbler may run several steps between dribbles.

11. Unless the dribbler is moving at great speed, he will usually have one step for each dribble taken.

The young player when dribbling must be cautioned to keep his head up. At first he may keep his eyes on the ball as he dribbles. However, he

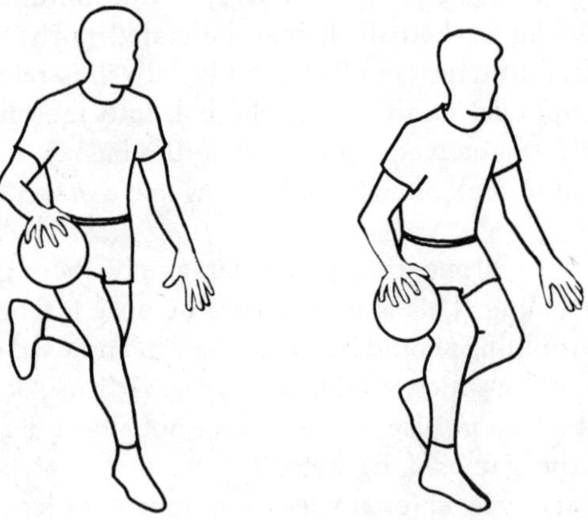

The high dribble with head up.

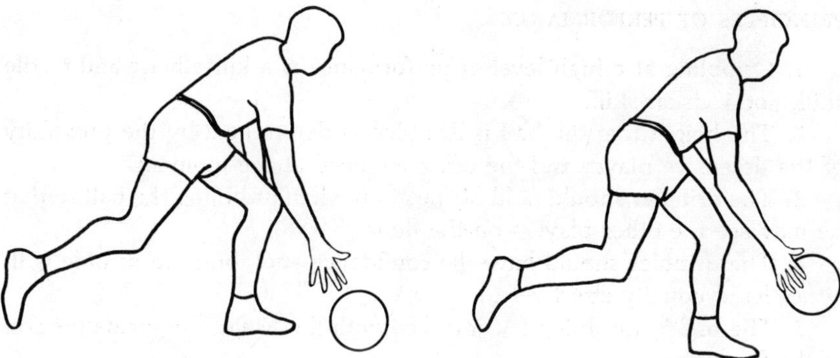

Finger tip control while dribbling.

must learn to dribble by the use of the touch system only, not by keeping his eyes on the ball. Dribbling by touch or feel should be developed with either hand from almost the very onset of basketball training. Many good basketball players have been eliminated from top flight competition because of their inability to dribble effectively with the non-preferred hand.

The young player should also be encouraged to execute the dribble by using only his fingers to produce the necessary force to bounce the ball the proper height from the floor. Finger control is the key to good dribbling. The dribbler may use his wrist and extension of the forearm to produce additional force if it is needed. This is because sometimes the force desired cannot be produced by the fingers alone.

The low controlled dribbled ball usually needs to be protected from the hands of a defensive player. Therefore, the stance of the dribbler is such

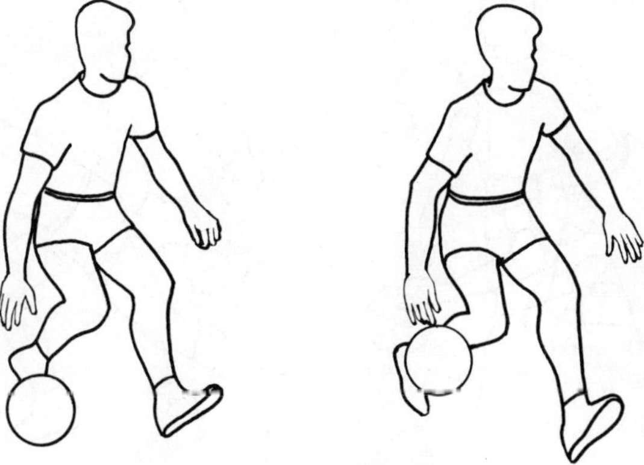

The low dribble.

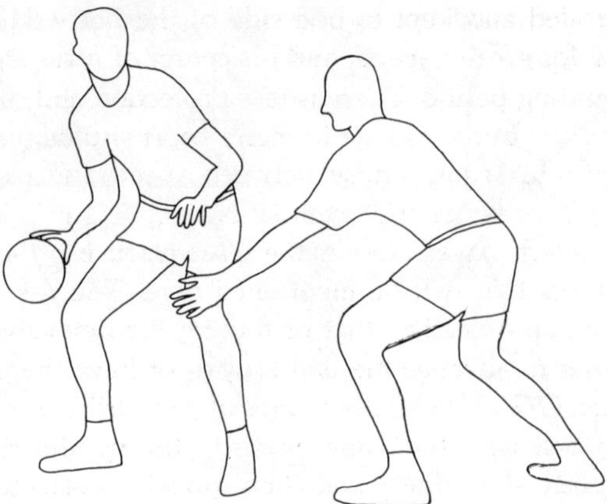

Protecting the dribble.

that he should not bend forward at the waist to get his hands down to the ball. Instead he should flex at the knees and lower his hips while keeping the trunk erect, thus giving the appearance of "sitting" while dribbling. There are two primary methods used in protecting the dribbled ball from a defensive player. One method is to bring the right foot forward, when dribbling with the right hand; to "hide" the ball behind a leg. The other method is to have the dribbler bring the opposite foot and hand forward, and to protect the ball behind this shield with his opposite leg. The dribbler is usually not effective attempting to protect the ball unless he also uses his free arm to aid in the protection.

When the offensive player wants to dribble with great speed, his body stance and his method of dribbling are quite different from the one described above. In this instance the ball is pushed far out in front of his body, rather

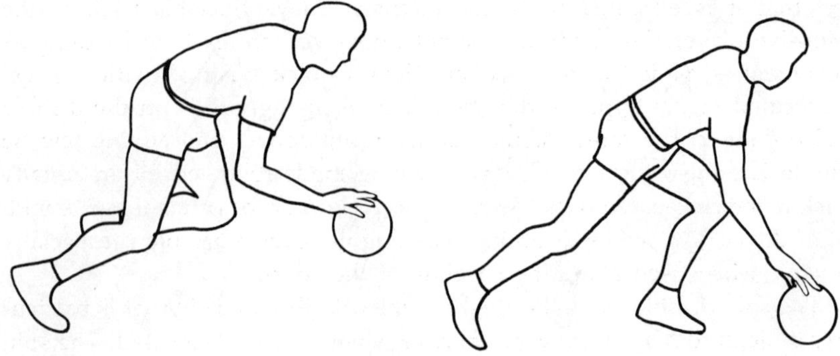

The fast dribble.

than being controlled and kept to one side of the body. His body stance is higher to allow for greater speed, and his center of mass is more forward during the accelerating period. There is less protection and control with the use of this procedure, but as is true in many sport situations, the offensive basketball player must compromise between speed and control to more effectively meet the needs of the given situation.

The highly skilled players can make effective use of some advanced dribbling procedures that will be mentioned here. The use of these techniques has a common objective, that of fooling the defensive player, thus freeing the dribbler to advance the ball toward or have the opportunity to shoot at the basket. One of these, the change of pace dribble, is accomplished by dribbling the ball with the same intensity throughout the movement, but having the body slow down and then quickly accelerate. The use of the drag dribble accomplishes the same purpose but directly opposite techniques are used. In the drag dribble, the player keeps moving at the same speed, but the ball slows down and speeds up during a given dribble, thus giving the appearance that the change of pace is taking place. These two techniques are often used when the player is driving down the sideline in an attempt to get a step ahead of the defensive player so that he can turn the corner and head toward the basket.

The cross-over dribble is executed by the dribbler stepping to the right in a dribbling motion. He plants the right foot then pushes off quickly to the left, while changing the ball in the dribble from the right hand to the left hand in front of his body. This changing of hands should be done by keeping the ball as low as possible with the left hand coming across to meet the bouncing ball. This skill, when executed properly, is virtually impossible to defend against because the defensive man must react to the first step taken to the right. Then, he has great difficulty recovering and changing his direction to keep up with the dribbler.

The single reverse dribble is quite similar to the cross-over dribble except that it is executed while the offensive player has his back to the defensive player. The body movements, however, are exactly the same. A movement is made in one direction, then a quick push-off with the feet is executed in the opposite direction. The changing hands on the dribble is also done in the same manner as described above. The double reverse dribble is done with a quick reverse being made followed by an equally quick reverse executed back toward the direction of the original movement. All of this is done while dribbling. The double reverse dribble is especially effective when used along the baseline of the court.

The spin dribble is another higher type of dribbling skill that is particularly difficult to master yet very effective when properly executed. The spin dribble is executed much in the same manner as the cross-over, yet with

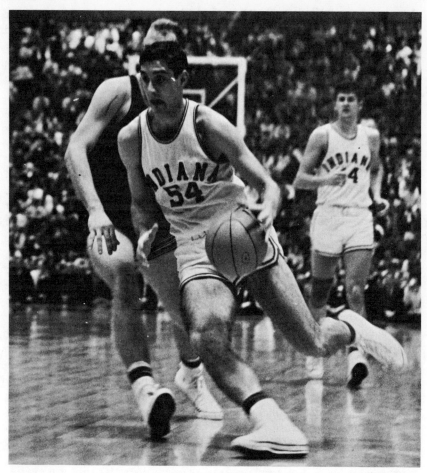

Making the sharp cut while dribbling.

a great deal less body movement. The idea behind its use is to give the appearance of starting in one direction but actually going in the other. This is accomplished by initiating the dribbled ball in one direction, but using a reverse spin that will bring the ball back toward the opposite direction. Once the ball returns to the dribbler he moves quickly in the direction of the reverse spin of the ball.

The use of the behind-the-back dribble is also very effective at times and should be encouraged as an upper level dribbling skill. However, its use should be quickly discouraged as a "showboat" tactic done by a player in a situation where it is not necessary. The behind-the-back dribble enables the dribbler to change direction without breaking stride. Also he does not have to worry about the ball being slapped away by a defender who is usually stationed just in front of him. More recently players have begun to use a dribble under one leg and recover with the opposite hand. These advanced procedures should be attempted only when the player has fully mastered the fundamental aspects of the dribbling skill.

The good dribbler reacts in his movements to defensive pressure. He should not follow any predetermined plan of advancing the ball. This is true also for the initiation of the dribble. Of course, if there is no pressure being made by the defender, the ball can merely be dropped in front of

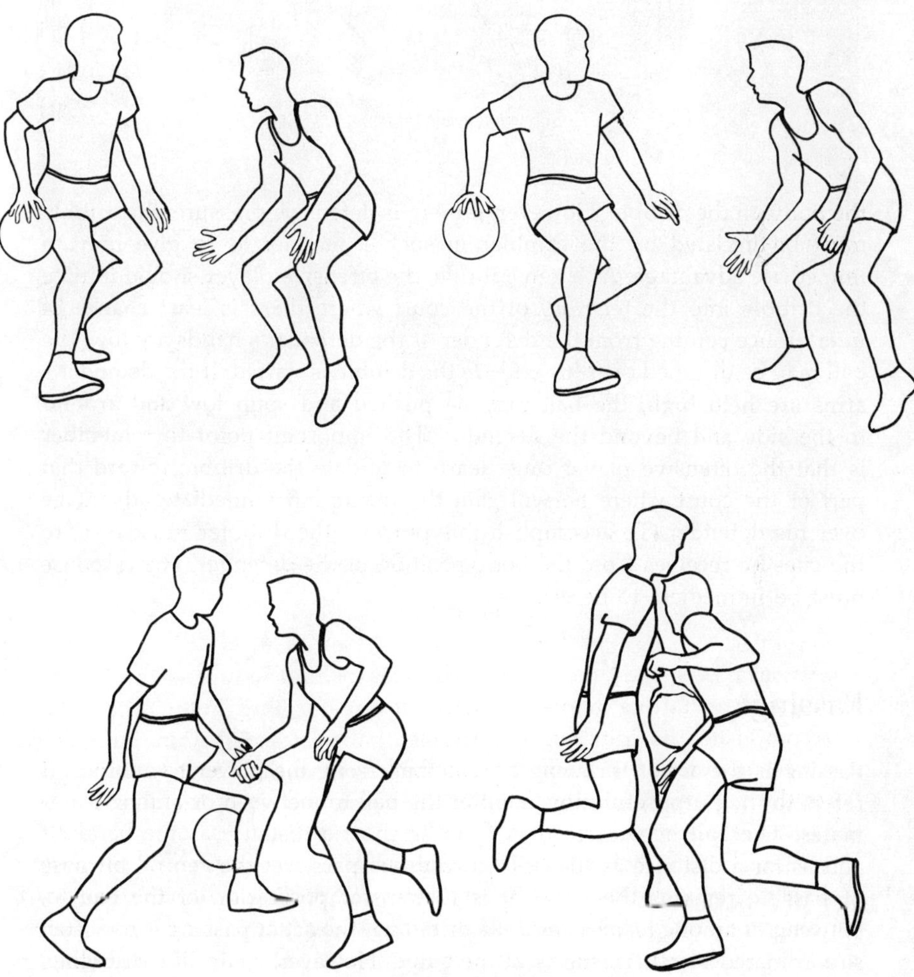

The behind the back dribble.

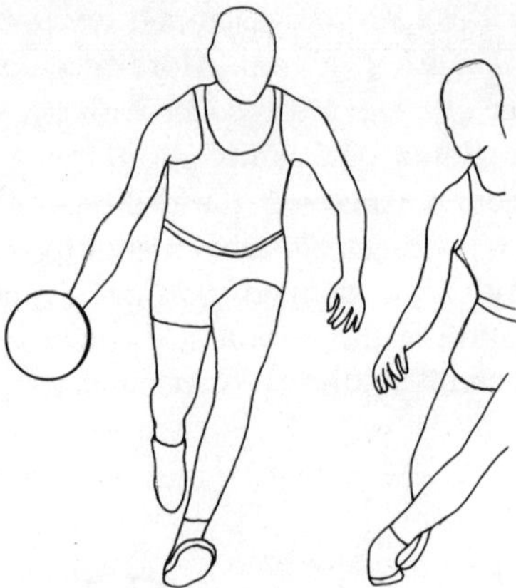

Protecting while cutting.

the body on the dribble. However, if there is defensive pressure, the dribble must be initiated by the dribbler in such a manner as to give him an immediate advantage. As a general rule, the offensive player should initiate the dribble into the territory of the court where there is least chance of interference coming from the defender. If the defender's hands are low, the ball may be dropped over his arms as the dribble is started. If the defender's arms are held high, the ball may be pushed and spun low and around to the side and beyond the defender. The important point to remember is that the offensive player must learn to initiate the dribble toward that part of the court where he will gain the maximum immediate advantage over his defender. To accomplish this purpose the dribbler must react to the cues he receives from the body position of the defender. His response must be immediate to be effective.

Passing

Passing is the act of throwing a basketball from one player to another. It refers to the purposeful movement of the ball to, between or among teammates. The ball may be thrown from as short a distance as the hand-off and as far a distance as the full-court length pass, yet the central purpose of passing remains the same. It is to transfer possession of the ball to, between or among teammates. Like dribbling, the act of passing is too often subordinated to other aspects of the game. However, again like dribbling, one would only need to observe critically players' performances in a basketball game to ascertain the contribution of passing t more important is the fact that many opportunitie tively are either lost or simply are never taken ad inadequate ability of some of the players to pass and at the strategically right moment.

PRINCIPLES OF PERFORMANCE

1. Good passers make optimum use of peripheral vision.
2. Except in unusual situations, passes should be executed so the ball is received at waist to chest high elevation from the floor.
3. Except in unusual situations, passes should be accomplished so the ball is delivered in as nearly horizontal plane as possible.
4. The vulnerable places available to pass the ball by a defensive player depends on the foot stance and hand positions of the defensive player.
5. The closer a defensive player is to the passer, the easier it is to pass the ball by him.
6. A passer must be able to pass the ball as quickly and as forcefully as possible from any position at which he receives it.
7. A definite target spot to pass to should be selected.
8. Knee extension, shoulder medial rotation, and forearm pronation contribute to the force of the ball when it is thrown.
9. The greater the velocity the ball attains, the more wrist and forearm pronation is utilized. Even knee extension may have been used.
10. The objective in passing is to get the ball to the desired teammate as quickly as possible without telegraphing the path of the ball to the defensive player. Crispness of delivery is essential.

The success of Bob Cousy, the former great Boston Celtic player in the professional ranks, bears witness to the high level of skill to which passing can be developed and to the tremendous impact that passing can make on the game as an offensive weapon. The good passer knows that if a ball is intercepted, it has been usually his throwing error that has resulted in the interception. The burden of responsibility for good passing being accomplished then must rest on the shoulders of the man who has thrown the ball, that is, the passer. The good passer, thus, must make use of peripheral vision. He may utilize the "distant stare" approach that tends to widen his peripheral vision field. He very seldom fixes his focus of attention on either his desired target or any player that is close in distance to him. The only way to take maximum advantage of offensive opportunities is for him to see as many things as possible. This makes it necessary for the passer to see as much of the offensive and defensive movement that occurs on the court as is possible from any particular spot on the floor.

s an unusual set of circumstances warrants the use of a lob pass, sser should deliver the ball with as much force as possible and as rly in a horizontal plane as is possible. The ball may be intercepted from e moment it leaves the passer's hands until it reaches the receiver's hands. The less time it takes for this transfer of the ball to take place, the less are the chances of an interception occurring. An effective pass is one that is delivered in a straight line which is the shortest distance between the point of release and the point of reception. This is, of course, most often a horizontal line. Among the major contributors to the force which propels the ball through space are knee extension, shoulder medial rotation, forearm pronation and wrist and finger extension. When time permits, the use of knee extension will add considerable force to the thrown ball especially in longer passes. Although, generally speaking, increased forearm pronation is the most important ingredient to use for increased force. This is especially true at those crucial times when the passer cannot afford to take the time to move into a bent knee passing stance before he passes the ball. The good passer is able to pass forcefully and accurately from many positions (including running at full speed). Quite often he has to throw the ball from the position in which he has received it. Under such circumstances the use of forearm pronation is the key to the increased force needed to make the pass a successful one.

Usually, the first and greatest problem that the passer encounters is attempting to pass the ball by his defensive man and have it on its way to the receiver. The procedure used to get the ball by the defensive man depends entirely on the position of the defensive player. How far away is he from the passer? What stance is he using? How are his hands placed? The instantaneous answers to these questions will provide the necessary information for the passer to use in initiating the passed ball through the most vulnerable areas around the defender. The closer in distance the defensive player is to the passer, the easier it is to pass the ball by him. The defensive player has to move his arms through a very wide arc to stop the pass if he is too close to the passer. An exception is when a defensive player is on "top" of the passer. This may be unsettling to the passer and it may be difficult to pass the ball. Moving away from the passer usually enables the defender to have time to make this arc of movement and increases his chances of intercepting the pass. Thus, the potential passer often dribbles toward the retreating defender to close the "gap." The passer should pick the most vulnerable area the defensive player offers him to pass the ball by him. For example, if the defensive player has his arms and hands down, the pass should be made over one of the defender's shoulders.

The vulnerable area will only remain so if the pass is not telegraphed. That is, the passer should look either at the floor or directly at the defensive man. In this way he cannot possibly telegraph his intensions to the opponents. The poor passer will usually sneak a quick look at his intended target (usually some part of his teammate's body) just before he passes the ball. This short look is usually just enough to tip off an alert defender and an interception may occur or the ball may be tapped away from its intended path.

Deception plays an important role in successful passing. Yet deception is a most often misunderstood concept especially by novice players. The novice player assumes that deception involves having the passer go through a number of complicated fakes before he passes the ball. The highly skilled passer does not rely on the use of many fakes to accomplish deception. The highly skilled passer usually achieves deception by (1) not telegraphing his intensions to the opponents, and (2) by passing the ball with great velocity. The novice player fails to recognize that the deception by the good passer is often created by the speed with which the ball is delivered to a teammate.

The preceding discussion applies to all types of passes used in the game of basketball. A detailed discussion of the various kinds of passes used by the good players would be repetitive. However some brief comments about selected passes will be made. The good passer uses the pass that is most needed in a particular situation. The two-hand chest pass is the one most frequently used by the players. The baseball pass, the hook pass, the two-hand overhead pass, the bounce pass and on occasion behind the back pass are also used quite often by the good passer. It should be noted that the bounce pass is perhaps the most misused of all the passes. The bounce pass violates the principle of passing the ball in as horizontal a path as

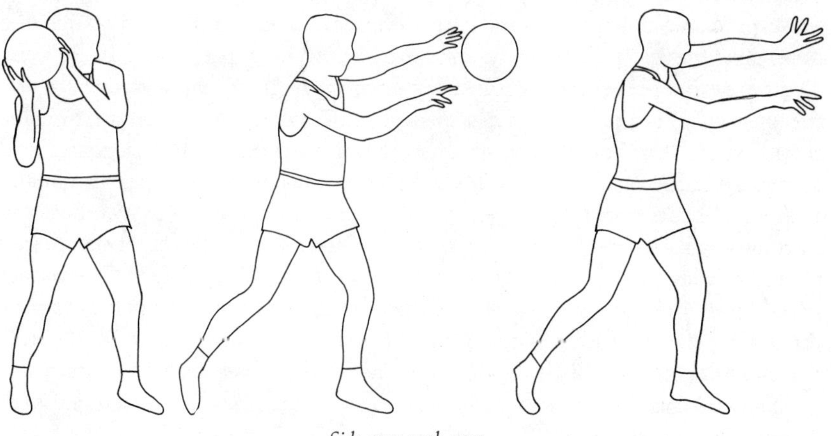

Side arm push pass.

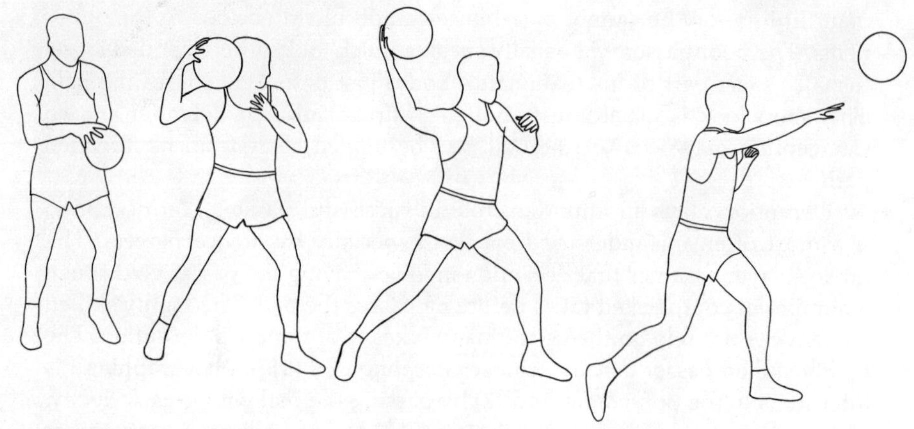

The baseball pass.

possible. Therefore, it should be used primarily by passers when they desire to pass only a short distance. Thus, this situation usually occurs in or near the basket. Also, they use it when they want the ball to go under the outstretched arms of a defender. When the path to a teammate is clear, there is no justification for using the bounce pass because the ball is traveling a slower rate to a teammate than if it were thrown so it traveled in the air.

Four abilities distinguish the highly skilled passer from the novice player. First, the highly skilled passer can throw the ball through a number of

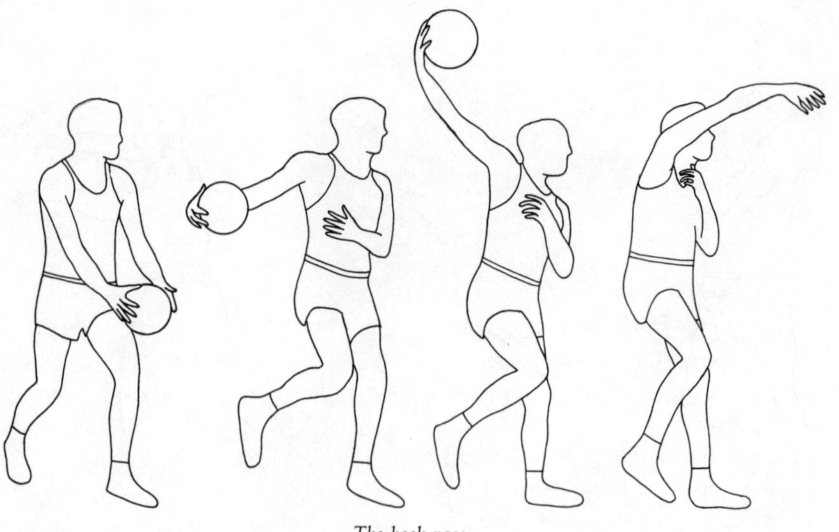

The hook pass.

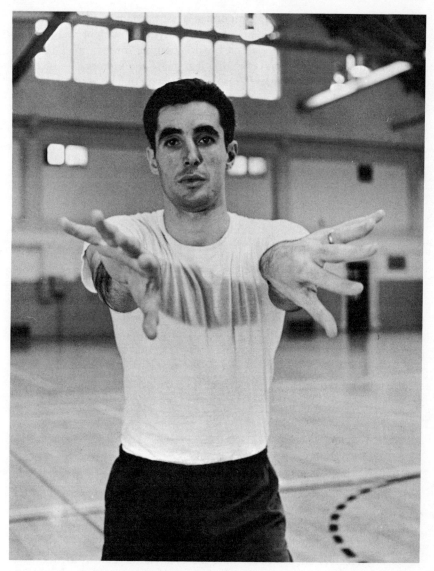

Pronation of hands shown in two-hand push pass.

defenders without it being intercepted. When extreme accuracy is necessary, and it often is not, the good passer exaggerates the pronated position of his forearms as he releases the ball so that the backs of his hands may come together as the follow through is completed. This enables the passer to maintain hand control on the ball for the fraction of a second longer than normal, thus, enabling him to pinpoint a pass. Second, the highly skilled passer is adept at passing from any position in which he might find himself when he has the ball. During a fast break situation, for example, a player must pass the ball down the court to a teammate the moment he receives the ball from another teammate. This means passing quickly and often from awkward positions. Third, perhaps what differentiates the good passer from the mediocre passer the most is the ability to pass the ball while moving quickly and at the same time be dribbling. This is especially noticeable in guard play when a team is fast breaking or dribbling during the offensive maneuvering spent in pattern play. In such situations the guard must deliver the ball to a teammate by a pass while he is in a dribbling movement (that is, he moves from a dribbling to a passing position virtually without pause). This skill is most difficult to master and should probably not be attempted by the young players, but possessing this ability is the hallmark of the highly skilled passer. Finally, he must be able to pass accurately on the run.

Receiving

Receiving is the act of gaining possession (catching) of a thrown ball from a teammate. While having a pass intercepted is definitely the fault of the passer, normally fumbling or bobbling a pass is the result of a miscue by a receiver. In football there is an old adage that states, "An end should be able to catch anything that he can touch." While this statement contains an obvious exaggeration, the general concept behind the adage is as worthy a goal for basketball as it is for football players. Certain catching principles are listed below:

PRINCIPLES OF PERFORMANCE OF CATCHING

1. Whenever possible the ball should be caught in front of the upper part of the receiver's body.
2. The gradual dissipation of force of a thrown ball is primarily accomplished by "giving" with the hands as the ball is received.
3. The receiver should never take his eyes off the ball in flight.
4. The hands should be in a thumbs-together position with the fingers pointing upward to receive a pass that is thrown above the waist.
5. The hands should be in a little-fingers-together position to receive a pass that is thrown below the waist.
6. When closely guarded, the receiver should catch the ball with the palm of one hand under and the palm of the other on top of the ball to prevent it from being slapped away by the defensive player.

A basketball player seldom merely catches a ball. Instead he usually must catch the ball, protect it, and continue to enter into the offensive movements of the team. If possible, the thrown ball should be received in front of the upper part of the body. This enables the receiver to have the best position for protecting the ball, to pass it on to a teammate, shoot at the basket, or dribble the ball in a given direction. In other words it is the most efficient position whereby the receiver may be able to maintain a variety of offensive responsibilities he had subsequent to receiving the ball. The receiver must dissipate the force of the ball by "giving" with his hands instead of with his trunk. This is because an offensive foul could easily be committed by the receiver who "gives" with his entire body to help dissipate the velocity of the ball.

The closely guarded receiver must protect the ball from the hands of his opponent. This is best done by either catching the ball from the hands in an over and under position, or the same results can be accomplished by immediately twisting the caught ball 90 degrees so that the hands are in the above mentioned position. The defensive player is most likely to slap at the underside of the ball and the hand and forearm of the receiver will protect the ball from this type of action.

The passer quite often creates deception by looking away from his intended receiver just as he passes the ball. On the other hand, the receiver must always maintain eye focus on the ball up to the moment before he catches it. It is relatively easy to pass accurately without looking at a target, but it is next to impossible to catch a basketball without watching it in its entire flight. This principle may be vividly and easily demonstrated to a team or a class by merely having them try to catch a pass while not looking at the ball in its flight.

The good receiver must "own" the territory in which he plans to receive the passed ball. He accomplishes this in two ways. One, he moves to meet the ball and establishes control of it as quickly as possible. Another way which is used especially by post players is to spread the legs and arms as wide as possible coupled with sticking out the buttocks toward the rear by bending at the waist. There movements are made just as the ball is being received. In effect, the territory into which the ball is thrown is protected from the opponents. The weakness in the use of this latter procedure is that the receiving position is not one in which quick movements can be made at the last moment to catch an off target pass.

The highly skilled player usually has mastered the skill of being able to turn a catch into a bounce or dribble when he is being harassed from all sides. This move may enable him to set a post position with the ball without difficulty. He should also be adept at using the over the shoulder type catch which is needed in fast break situations. This is a most difficult catch to make because the player is moving quickly and must frequently convert the passed ball into a dribble before he commits a traveling violation.

Shooting

Shooting may be defined as the act of propelling the ball toward the goal in a type of throwing motion with the use of one or two hands. This general, simplified definition conveys to the reader neither the importance of such a movement nor the extreme difficulty of being able to reach a high level of performance in the execution of the act. Generally speaking, shooting is the most important and the most difficult skill to master in the game of basketball. In the following presentation the term shooting is meant to imply the execution of the action in a game situation, that is, under competitive pressure. Many young men have become extremely adept as good shooters in practice, but exhibit very mediocre shooting performance in competitive game situations.

There are many different shots that have been and are used in the game of basketball. Also, there are many variations in styles of execution used for each shot. It is believed that a good shooter is one who can virtually shoot from any stance with the use of any shooting style if he finds it necessary to do so.

There are also many ways to teach shooting. The methods and styles that are considered to be best for teaching most basketball players how to shoot properly are presented here. Selected principles of performance in shooting are brought up for consideration before detailed discussion is conducted.

PRINCIPLES OF PERFORMANCE

1. Good shooters should always aim at a specific target.
2. Good shooters should maintain constant eye focus on the target until the ball is released.
3. The ball should always be "wiggled" just before the release is begun in order to have good touch in shooting.
4. The shooter should not hold his body in a fixed position for a very long time before releasing the ball (especially his arms and hands).
5. The ball should be delivered with a reverse spin in most instances.
6. The better the shooter, the more intense is the concentration on the act of shooting. Also he does not "spray" his shots. His missed shots are either long or short, not right or left.
7. Shooting is characterized by medial shoulder rotation, elbow extension, forearm pronation, and wrist flexion.
8. The longer the distance from the basket the ball is delivered, the more pronounced is the forearm pronation.
9. The longer shots require that the ball be released at a higher angle (greater arch).

10. Longer shots require that parts of the body be used to add momentum to the hand.

11. Technically, the higher the arch of the shot, the more chance it has to go in the basket.

12. A 45 degree angle of release enables the player to propel the ball the longest distance.

13. Shots released at a greater height from the floor need to be released with less arch.

14. Most shots should be aimed at a target (spot) just over the rim.

15. Every player must be able to rebound the ball off the board into the basket as he gets close to the basket.

16. Right hand one hand set shots should normally be delivered with the right foot forward.

17. The more spin that is given to the ball, the further from the basket it can be rebounded off of the board.

18. The non-shooting hand should be used to support the ball until the last moment before release of the ball occurs. However, the shooter should be careful not to "thumb" the ball with the non-shooting hand.

19. As a player moves up in competitive level, he must be able to deliver his shots with greater quickness in order to have greater opportunity to achieve success in scoring.

20. While there are many styles of shooting a ball at the basket, it appears that there are certain basic patterns of mechanics that underlie all good shooting styles.

Good shooters always aim at a *specific target,* and they concentrate on hitting that target to the exclusion of all other things (extraneous sounds and movements). More than anything else the exhibition of these two characteristics, aim and concentration, helps distinguish the good shooter from the average shooter. Today most players aim at a spot just over the front of the rim. They do so for two very good reasons. First, when one aims at a spot just over the front of the rim, one does not have to change the target point when moving about on the floor, and this enables the shooter to always have the opportunity to aim at the same spot. Second, glass backboards do not make a good target to aim at, especially when there are people located in the stands behind them. To select a clearly defined target on the backboard would be very difficult to do in a brightly lit gymnasium where fans are permitted to sit in the sections at the ends of the playing floor. The spot just over the front of the rim then becomes the most logical target under these circumstances. However, some coaches advocate that shooting at the back edge of the rim will bring the best results. This is sometimes true because shots usually stray a certain amount in either direction from the intended target. If this target is the back edge of the rim, then they (coaches) contend that the slightly short shot will still have a chance to get over the front edge of the rim and into the basket. On the other hand, the slightly long shot will have a chance to rebound into the basket off the backboard. If a tense shooter aims at just over the front edge of the rim, his slightly short shot will hit the front of the rim and fall short. Shooting at the back edge of the rim then seems to be the best target for the tense shooter to use especially during the early part of the game.

It seems to be very helpful for the player to *wiggle* the ball slightly while it is in his hands and just before he delivers it toward the basket. This preliminary *wiggle* made by the performer is quite similar in nature to that done in many other sport skills such as in golf and in baseball batting. The *wiggle,* or "waggle" as it is called in golf, seems to help decrease tension and enables the performer to have a better feel of the object. Perhaps just as importantly, the wiggle seems to initiate the rhythm of the movement that is so necessary to successful performances in sports.

The shooting position should never be held for too long a time before the ball is released. This over-delaying action seems to allow tension to build up, destroys the rhythm and seemingly "freezes" the performer. The most probable explanation of this phenomenon is that holding the ball in any kind of static position for too long a period of time probably causes neuromuscular firing to occur on both sides of the arm lever therefore creating the tenseness in it. Thus, freezing or choking of the performer occurs.

The importance of concentration in the development of good shooting skill has been mentioned previously, but it bears repeating. Concentration means being able to "shut out" the crowd noises, opponent noises and all the many movements that the player picks up in the periphery of his vision and hearing. Concentration also means zeroing in on the point of aim and delivering the shot with singlemindedness and assurance. Most likely the main difference between the "three o'clock" good shooter and the "eight o'clock" good shooter lies in the degree of concentration. The "three o'clock" shooter cannot concentrate at the later time under the pressure of the "eight o'clock" game situations. It is a moot point as to the extent to which this kind of concentration can be developed by a boy who has already reached the senior high school level. If it can be learned, it can only be learned if the eight o'clock situation is recreated as many times as possible during the practice periods. It can be stated that the extent to which it is possible to learn or acquire a high degree of concentration is most likely related to the number of exposures during practice which a player has had that are game-like in nature.

Shooting in basketball falls under the general category of throwing, and therefore the player exhibits many of the characteristics that are seen during all throws. For example, the ball is released off the inside tips of the first two fingers and is delivered with a reverse spin toward the shooter. The shot is characterized by the player having medial shoulder rotation, elbow extension, forearm pronation, and wrist flexion. The pronation factor is probably not as significant as in other types of throws especially in connection with shots, but pronation will become more pronounced as the shooter gets farther and farther away from the basket. Longer shots also require that more body parts are in action to add momentum to the shooting hand. The good long-shooter steps into the shot with his entire body, moves his hips with him, starts the ball from a lower position, and makes more use of knee extension when delivering the ball toward the basket. The ball is moved through a greater distance before release takes place thus allowing more time for force to be built up. The follow through from the execution of this type of shot is also much more pronounced than when shooting a short shot. This is due to the greater force that is generated and also because the hand stays against the ball slightly longer allowing for a slightly longer time period over which the force is applied. These above mentioned actions, done to exert greater force during the longer distance shot, are equally applicable to the long jump shot as they are to the long set shot. In principle it is possible to shoot the ball a much longer distance when the feet maintain contact with the floor until the moment of release takes place than if the player is in the air and releases the ball.

The flight of any ball follows a parabolic path. Theoretically, this means that the higher the angle of flight, the more chance the ball has to go through the basket. Equally important, though, to the success of the shooter are the softness with which the ball strikes the rim and the amount of spin imparted to the ball at release. In order to have both softness and control, most shots are delivered with a very medium arch. However, long shots are most advantageously released at any angle of near 45 degrees. This high angle of release allows the player to make the most efficient use of force.

Another important facet in shooting is the relationship of the height of the body and ball release position to the angle of flight of the ball. This in turn is related to the amount of force that is needed to get the ball into the basket. Shooting the ball up in the air against gravity is what requires a great deal of force, and the higher the release position the less effect the force of gravity will have on its flight. During the early history of basketball a 6-foot tall guard shooting a two hand set shot probably had the ball reach a release height of just over 6 feet. Thus, in order to develop enough lifting force to put the ball into the 10-foot tall basket the ball had to travel a good distance against the force of gravity. Today, a 6 foot 5 inch player shooting a jump shot probably has the ball reach a height of almost 9 feet 6 inches at the point of release. Therefore, the shot does not need nearly as great a lift in order to go into the basket. It does not have to go against the force of gravity nearly as long as did the 6 foot shooter's shot. This means that the modern jump shooter actually has to use much less force in his short shots and therefore can get more softness and touch in his shooting. This is one of the most important factors in determining the difference in the shooting abilities of today's players as compared with those of past years. The answer lies in a purely mechanical concept, yet it is often misunderstood, particularly in "cracker barrel" arguments concerning the relative merits of today's players as opposed to those of the past. The fact is that the 6 foot 6 inch or taller jumping jack forward of today comes very close to being able to shoot his jump shot down rather than up at the basket. In terms of the laws of physics and mechanics, he actually performs his physical task with less force than did the set shooter of years ago. However, the two-hand set shooter since he used both hands could shoot the ball from a farther distance with greater accuracy.

While it is true that the vast majority of shooters today aim at a target just over the front of the rim for most of their shots, it is no less true that every good shooter should be able to use the backboard as a target in some of his shots, especially as he gets close to the basket. In this instance the shooter must have a proper concept of the spin that he puts on the ball at release and the way in which the spin behaves as it hits the backboard. The more spin that is put on the ball, the farther away from the rim it can be placed on the board. The giant centers playing on defense today often cause the shooter to have to shoot over a long pair of outstretched arms when he is close to the basket. To avoid having the shot blocked in this situation the shooter must sometimes lay the ball very high up on the board with sufficient spin on it to cause it to rebound toward the basket.

The non-shooting hand should be used to support the ball until the last moment before the shot is released. The practice of keeping this hand on the ball until the last moment seems to be characteristic of all good shooters. Some prefer to have the non-shooting hand on the side of the ball, while others prefer to have it in front of the ball and opposite the shooting hand. Whichever technique is chosen, this practice will add to the balance and control with which the shot can be delivered, and thus will improve the accuracy of the shot.

As a player moves up the competitive ladder, quickness in delivering his shots becomes an important factor in his success as a shooter. Many players are good shooters when given ample time to execute the shot, but these players miss opportunities to shoot because they lack the necessary quickness to deliver the ball and execute the shooting act with great speed. This tends to diminish their effectiveness as shooters. This is an important factor to remember in planning shooting practices. Effort should be made to insure that shooting in practice is executed with the same quickness that would be required in the game situation.

It has been suggested here that there are many styles of shooting, and this is certainly true. Nevertheless, one can point to a basic pattern of shooting that appears to be the "best" pattern, and the pattern that is exhibited by most of the great shooters. This pattern would involve such things as aiming at a specific target, constant eye focus, a relaxed stance, adequate concentration, support of the ball with the non-shooting hand, elbow of the shooting arm pointed directly in line with the basket, quickness in executing the shot, and desire to score. A description of some of the basic shots is contained in the subsequent pages.

ONE-HAND SET SHOT

The right hand shooter will most often shoot the one-hand set shot with the right foot placed forward of the left. This position helps fix the mass

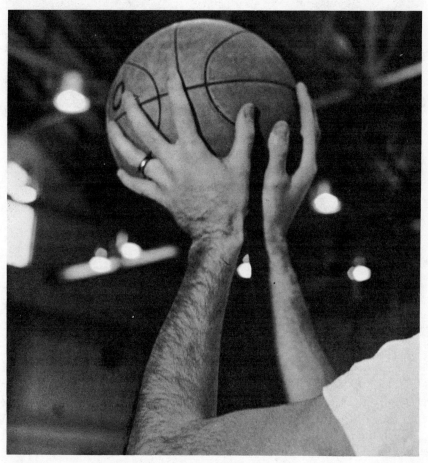

One grip used in shooting one-hand set shots (#1).

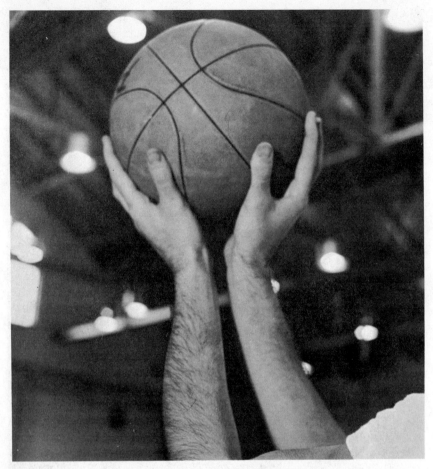

One grip used in shooting one-hand set shots (# II).

of the body so that the least amount of body motion occurs to interfere with the shooting action. The ball is held in the fingers, with the first finger and thumb of the shooting hand forming a "V." The ball is grasped slightly off center to its right by a right-handed shooter. The head of the shooter must be held still and the best use made of the dominant sighting eye. This will mean that a right-eyed shooter will want to turn his head slightly to the left or right so that the dominant eye can have the best position for sighting the target. The shot is initiated by the ball being dropped slightly to establish rhythm, utilize gravity, and provide greater distance through which the force may be applied to the ball. The wiggle has preceded this dropping action and aids in establishing the rhythm of the movement and

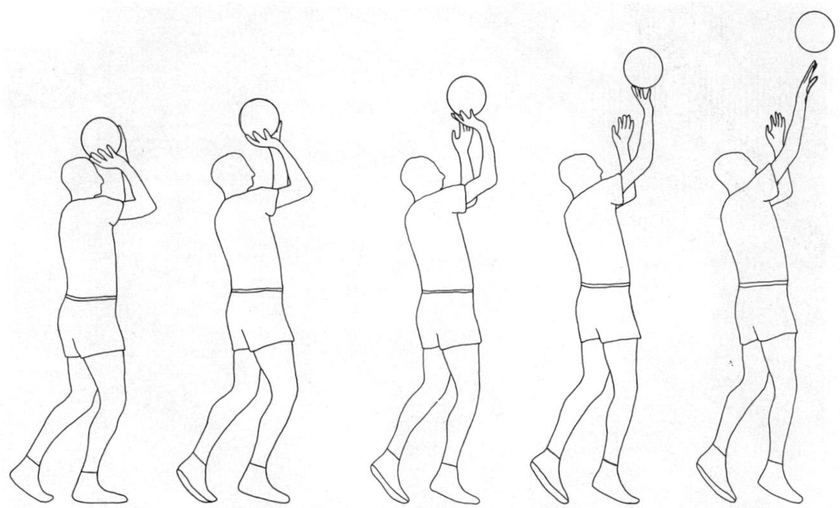

Executing the one-hand set shot.

gives the player the proper feel of the ball. The shot is begun somewhere between chest and shoulder height and the ball may be dropped almost to hip height before the upward movement of the arm is begun. However, the higher the ball is held, the less apt it is to be blocked by an opponent. The ball is brought up slightly off center of the front of the body and along the side of the head. In this way the vision is never obstructed and the shooter can maintain constant eye focus on the target. As the ball is brought up the elbow comes up too and is pointed directly in line with the target. As the ball is moved toward the release it actually becomes a one-hand shot because the other hand that has acted as a balancer is taken off the ball at this point. The ball is released with finger control, a gentle snap of the wrist, and a smooth arm follow-through. The ball is flipped, not pushed, as it is released. The ball is released by action from the first two fingers, giving it a reverse backspin. Depending on how long a distance the shooter is attempting to propel the ball, the follow-through position may find him well up on his toes, and he may even have to make a short jump after the release if he has delivered a set shot from a long distance.

TWO-HAND SET SHOT

The two-hand set shot is used in the same situations in which the one-hand set shot is used except in modern basketball it is used by only a few players who desire to shoot a very long distance. The ball is held in the fingers with the hands nearly equally distributed on it. The ball is

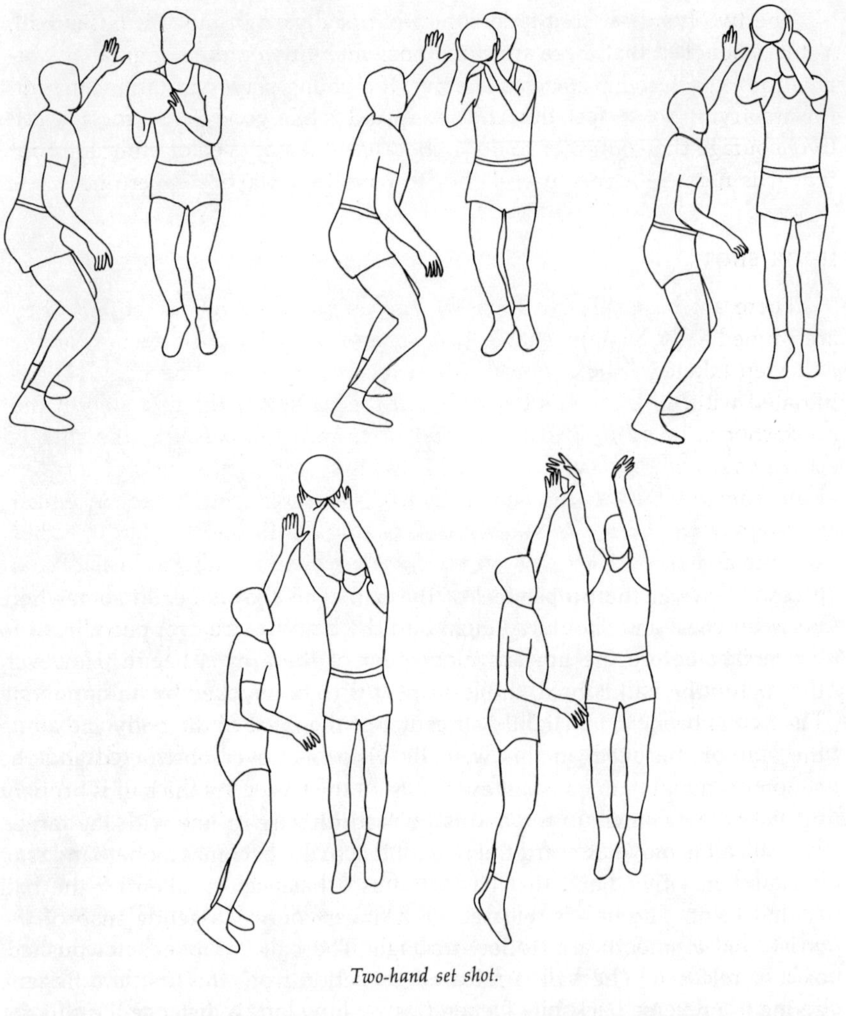

Two-hand set shot.

held somewhere between waist and chest height which is a somewhat lower starting position than that used in the one-hand set shot. After the wiggle the ball is dropped to start the rhythm of the shooting motion and to create a greater distance through which the throwing force is applied. The farther out the shooter is from the basket, the lower the starting position of the ball. Eye focus is constantly maintained on the target, as the upward movement of the ball is so fast the target is never lost during this phase. The ball is propelled toward the basket in such a manner that the arms and hands are pronated. The spin and follow-through are very similar in nature to that found in the one-hand shot, and, in fact, in the two-hand set shot one of the hands actually comes off the ball a little sooner than the other.

The two-hand set shot is in somewhat of disuse in modern basketball. Yet it is believed that there are situations where it would be of great advantage for a coach to have such a shooter. If a young player has an inclination toward trying to perfect this shot, it would make good sense for a coach to encourage the youngster to do so. Because it is not used often is no proof that it is not still a very useful shot to have in a player's repertoire.

HOOK SHOT

There are basically two types of hook shots used in basketball. They are immediately distinguishable from one another by the direction of the first step taken by the shooter as he executes the shot. The hook shot is initiated with the shooter's back toward the basket. If the first step of the hook shot is taken toward the basket or toward the baseline, the shot is actually a driving type of pivot shot. If the first step by the shooter is taken away from the basket, the shot becomes a sweeping hook shot in which closeness to the basket is not of primary concern to the shooter. In either case, the actual mechanics of the shot itself are very similar (in each type) and may be treated as one shot. Some big people are able to shoot a hook shot with only slight movement of the feet. They then usually use less of a sweeping motion with the arms.

The shot is initiated by taking one step that is usually a very long step. This accomplishes the dual purpose of momentarily freeing the shooter from his defensive man and also providing the beginning rhythm for and impetus to the movement. The ball is started quite low with the hip away from the defensive player acting as a shelve or cover below which the ball is protected. The ball rests in the fingers much in the same manner as is done in the one hand set shot but from an underneath cup position. As the shot is brought up alongside the right hip, the left shoulder is turned to the left and the head is turned in the same direction, that is, toward the basket in order to maintain eye focus on the target. As the ball is brought up near shoulder height the shooting arm becomes almost fully extended, and the left hand leaves the ball and moves downward. This provides additional neuromuscular facilitation for the movement of the right arm farther upward and adds additional force to the ball. The ball is released off the fingertips with the first two fingers giving the final impetus to the ball. During the follow-through the right hip completes its rotation and the first finger of the right hand ends up pointing directly at the target. The shooting arm is pronated as in other shots. The ball in the execution of the hook shot is released with reverse backspin, and is usually released at a flatter angle than in the set shot. Hook shooters quite often use a spot on the backboard as their target. (However, some aim at the basket.) This is done for two reasons. First, the flatter shot has more success if it caroms into the basket

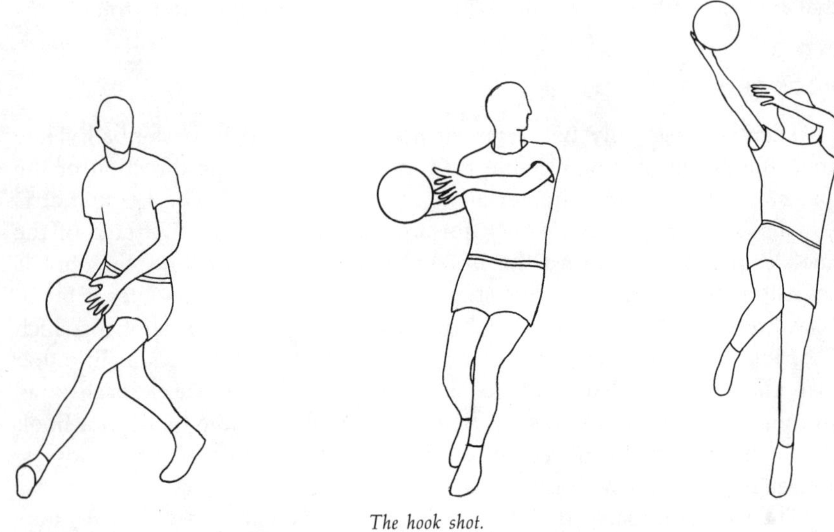

The hook shot.

off the backboard, and second, the shot is often taken from an angle to one side of the basket which lends itself to the use of the backboard. Some hook shooters, particularly those of the step-away sweeping variety, use a higher arc and aim the ball directly at the basket, but this seems to be a more difficult shot to master.

In recent years the hook shot has been used more and more by guards and forwards when they are driving toward the basket. The presence of a very tall center on defense makes it almost impossible for them to be able to drive all the way into the basket and get an unmolested lay-up. So, more and more guards and forwards have begun to use short hook shots to get the ball over the outstretched arms of the taller defenders. The execution of this shot is essentially done in the same manner as is done in the pivot hook shot.

JUMP SHOT

Today, the most important offensive weapon in basketball is the jump shot. No offensive maneuver has so completely dominated the game as the

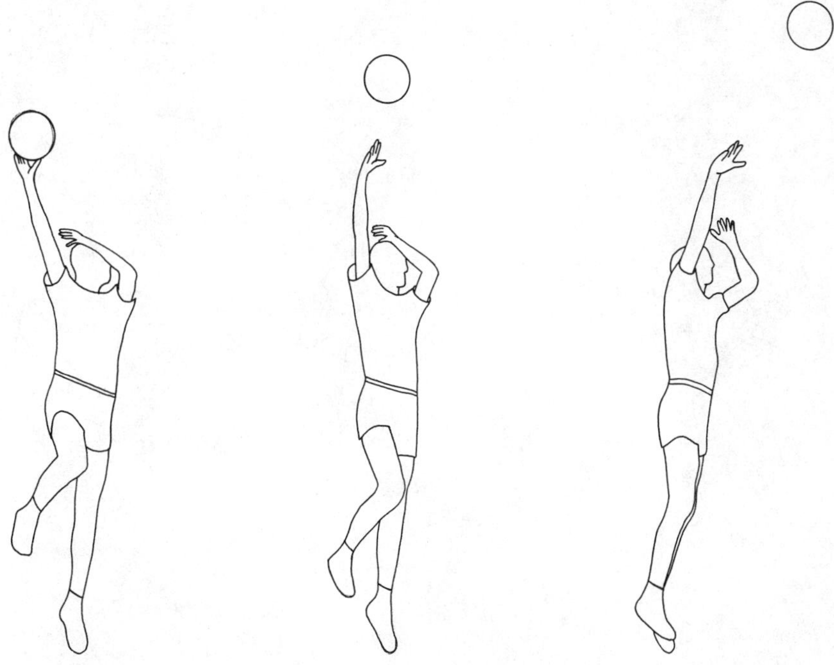

jump shot has done in recent years. The jump shot is used by almost all players shooting from all angles and from almost any distance. It has tended virtually to eliminate the use of the set shot. In terms of mechanics, the jump shot is remarkably similar to that of the set shot, and it is probably correct to state that the jump shot is a set shot made by a player in the air after he has jumped. Since the set shot has already been presented, only those aspects of the jump shot that are somewhat different from that of the set shot will be discussed.

The jump shooter must set himself in the air before he shoots. As he gathers himself for the jump his feet should be directly underneath his body. Plantar flexion of the foot and knee extension provide the primary force thrusting him upward. These movements are aided by the ball being brought up as the jump is made. The ball is held in exactly the same manner as that used in the set shot. The ball is brought up for the shot along the front of the body, but somewhat off center; again, as is done in the set shot. The position of the elbow seems to be the one fundamental aspect of the mechanics of the jump shot movement that cannot be violated and have the player be effective. The elbow is brought up higher than in the set shot

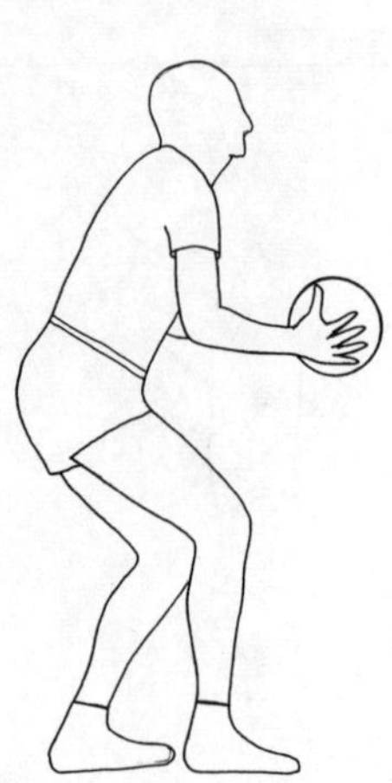
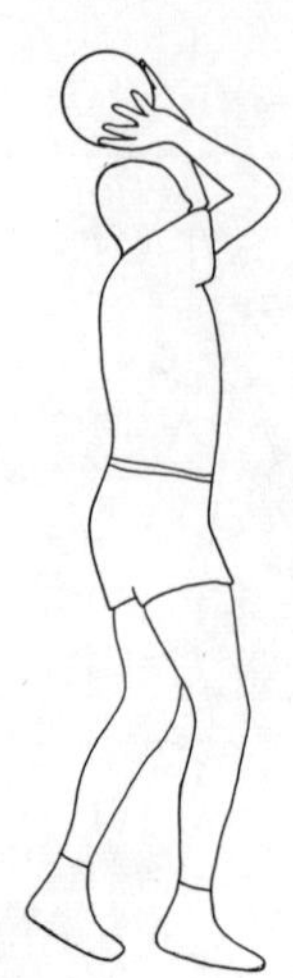
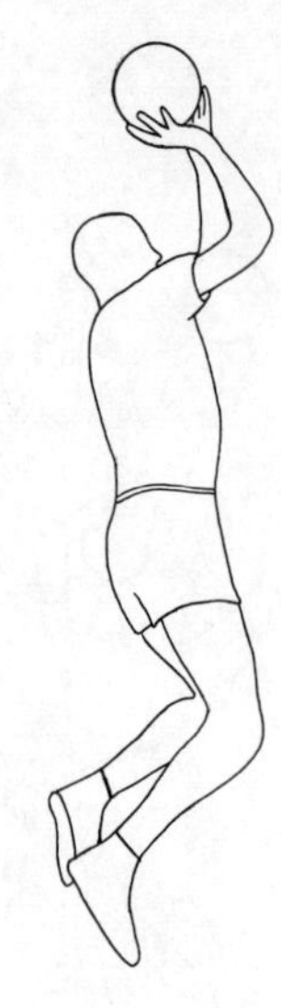

The jump shot.

and the ball is brought back farther behind the head or to the side of the head than is done in the set shot. The elbow is pointed directly in line with the target, and any violation of this position seems to completely eliminate the possibility of the shooter being successful. Most players release the ball at the height of their jump, but some players release the ball slightly after the apex of the jump has been reached. Therefore, they give the impression of "hanging" in the air. The jump shot has less arch on the ball than in the set shot because it is not possible for the player to exert as much force as can be exerted when foot contact is maintained with the floor. Yet because the jump shot is released from a position higher from the floor than is the set shot, the ball is less affected by gravity. The jump shot often requires a great deal less force to be exerted by the shooter at release than is true in the set shot taken from the same floor distance.

The jump shooter may jump almost to his maximum jumping height or he may use a quick short jump before delivering the ball depending upon the situation. Usually the jump shooter tends to jump higher the closer he is to the basket. This is usually done because defensive pressure is usually tougher and tighter as the player gets closer to the basket and the ball has

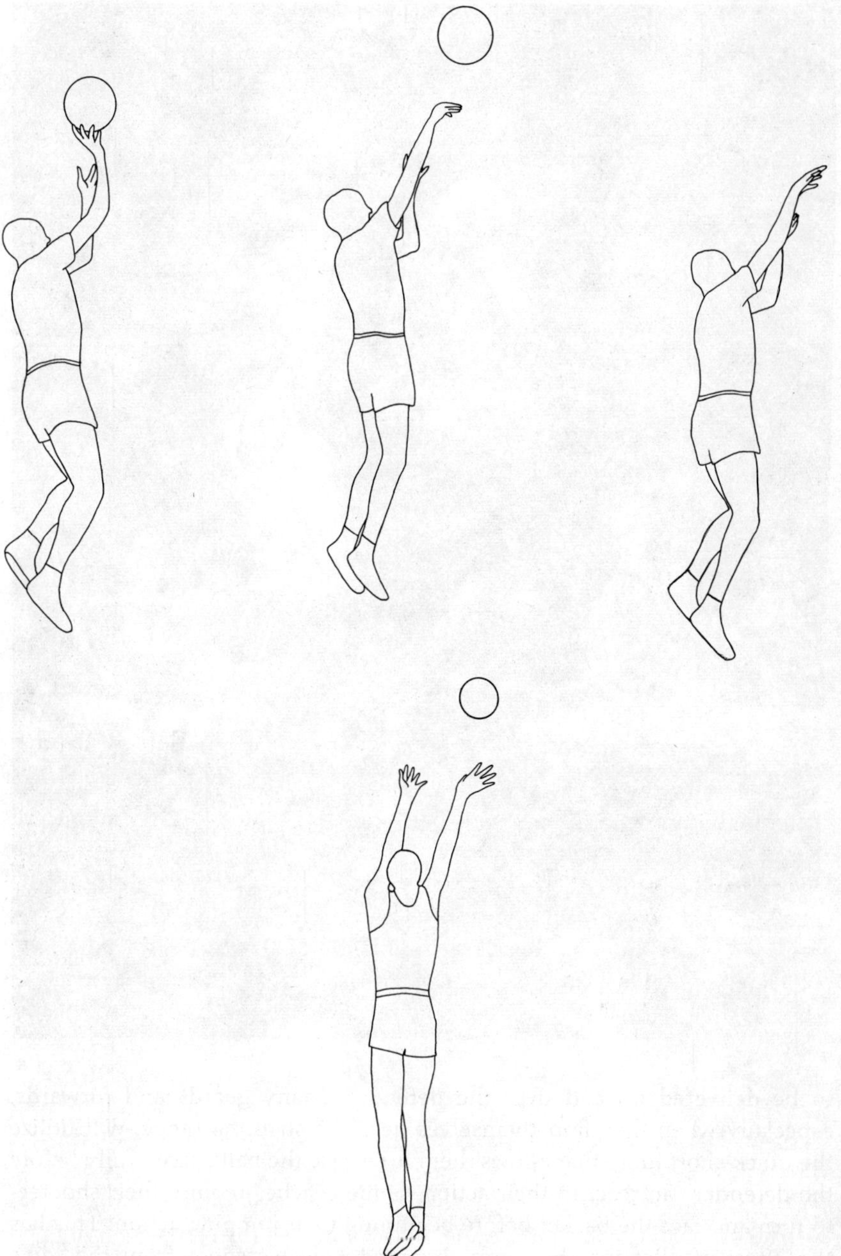

Jump shot showing the extent of left hand contact with ball.

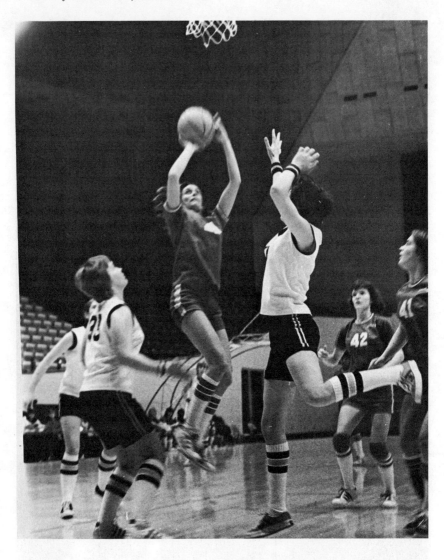

to be delivered up and over the defender. Many guards and forwards, especially when they find themselves near the shooting range, will utilize the quick short jump that allows them to release the ball successfully before the defender can react to their action. Some coaches require their shooters to turn and face the basket before beginning their jumping action. This has the effect of allowing the jump shooter to always shoot from the same position no matter whether he has been moving in a direction to the left or to the right. If the player jumps and shoots without making this turn,

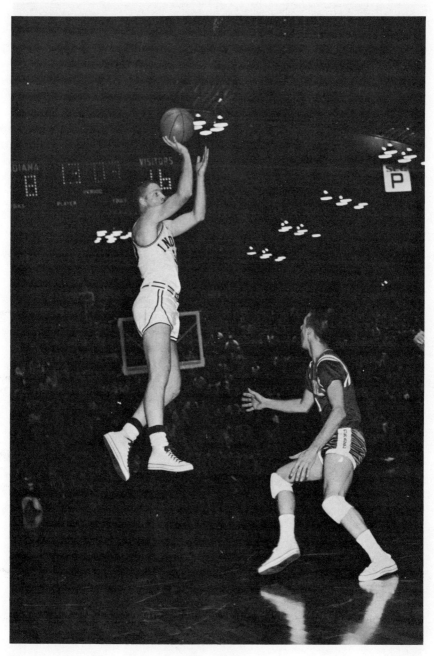

Maximum jump is made by shooter.

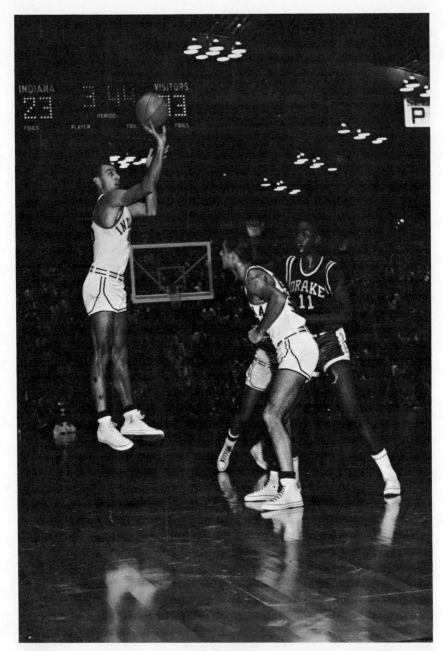

Eye is kept on target.

then the jump shot moving to the right will be somewhat different from that of the jump shot made while moving to the left. This will be true because the movements made in gathering for the jump, protecting the ball, and bringing the ball up for the shot will be somewhat different, executed from the one specific side rather than from the front. Once the ball is brought up into shooting position, however, the rest of the mechanics of the action are identical.

The jump shooter probably experiences more difficulty maintaining eye focus on the target than does any other type of shooter. There is a tendency for the novice to look down at the ball as he gathers for the jump. This will cause him to lose sight of the target. It cannot be emphasized too much that concentration on the target is the key to success in jump and all shooting. Constant eye focus on the target while preparing for and during the execution of the shot seems to be one of the important characteristics of the good shooter. The jump shooter must be cautioned to keep his head up during all phases of the jumping movement. If he does this, it will become quite natural for him to keep his eye focused on the target.

LAY-UP

The term "lay-up" applies to a wide range of so called short shots made by a player while in a running stride and when close to the basket. These include the wholly unmolested "dog shot" or "cripple," which is quite likely the easiest two points received by the players in basketball. The driving lay-up, however, is perhaps the most difficult shot to make in basketball, especially when a tall defender provides defensive harassment as the shooter draws close to the basket. The mechanics involved in the execution of these different types of lay-ups are remarkably similar, even though the degree of difficulty varies. A thorough understanding and effective use of the proper mechanics of executing the lay-up shot may aid considerably in lessening the difficulty in accomplishing the lay-up shots.

The lay-up is a running shot and the last stride made by the player just before the shot is taken should be a longer one. The leap or jump of the lay-up should be upward and not outward. It is an error to jump outward. This action causes the execution of many driving lay-ups to be much more difficult than they need to be. Utilization of the knowledge that horizontal momentum must be converted into vertical height can go a long way toward helping to eliminate this error. As the longer last stride is being taken the shooter should lean backward. Without first making this backward lean it is virtually impossible for the player to jump vertically from a run. Most shooters take off on the foot opposite their shooting hand because this is the most natural movement. It also will enable the player to attain the highest jump because the most efficient use is made of the momentum that has been built up during the run that has preceded the shooting of the lay-up shot.

However, there are players who prefer to take off on the foot on the same side of their body as their shooting hand. While this technique will not allow as high a jump to be accomplished, it will help insure that the jump is as directly vertical as possible because the use of the foot on the same side as the shooting hand will in effect serve as a braking action and help the player convert horizontal velocity to vertical lift.

Once players attain a fairly high level of skill they might experiment with the use of both techniques to find out the one that best suits their style of play. Regardless of which foot is used as the takeoff, once the jump is initiated the mechanics of movement are exactly the same for either method. The shooter must be cautioned as mentioned to attempt to make his jump upward instead of outward as he goes in for the lay-up. One good method of making players conscious of doing this phase of the lay-up correctly is to have them measure the horizontal distance from their takeoff to their landing. If their jump has been vertical, the distance will not be too great, but if they have been making much of a jump outward instead of upward, this distance will be significantly greater. If the shooter wants to add height to his jump in the lay-up, his free leg should be flexed at the knee and brought vigorously upward toward the waist at the takeoff of the jump. Adding impetus to the height can also be gained from a vigorous upward thrust of the ball at the takeoff. This is also a good move to use from the standpoint of overcoming and breaking through any defenders that may be there to attempt to block the lay-up shot of the shooter on his way up.

There are two basic styles of shooting the lay-up, and the use of either one is largely an individual and/or a situational matter. One style is to hold the ball much in the same manner as is done in a one-hand set shot, that is actually to shoot the ball against the backboard with an overhand motion. The other style is to release the ball with an underhand motion. Regardless of the one used, it is good procedure to always use the backboard as a target in lay-up shots. Both hands are always kept on the ball until just before it is released.

Novices should learn to shoot lay-up shots from either side of the basket using the left hand on the left side of the basket and the right hand on the right side. In a right-handed lay-up shot attempted from the left side of the basket the ball is always in danger of hitting the left side of the rim as it moves upward. Also it is much more likely to be blocked by defensive players because this movement cannot be as easily protected with the body as one made with the left hand. The right-handed lay-up from the right side of the basket is a protected shot.

At higher levels of skill the lay-up shot must be executed with some degree of deception and finesse. For example, the good driving lay-up shooter should be able to shoot a hook lay-up, a reverse lay-up, and a spinning lay-up shot. He should be able to execute these shots sometimes as he turns his head to look squarely at the defensive player. Often a small player will have to lay the ball rather high on the board and farther away from the basket than he would if he were taller or unmolested. This move requires that a great deal of spin be imparted to the ball at release so that it will hit the board and, by virtue of the spin, bounce at the low angle into the basket.

Time devoted to shooting lay-ups is often wasted during a practice session. This is true not because these shots do not need to be practiced as much as others, but because the players merely form two lines and drive in at their leisure to shoot an unmolested lay-up. This will not help improve their shooting skill in game situations. In order to have the lay-up shooting practice be effective the shooter should be moving in practice at the same speed in which he is likely to be moving during a game. He should face the same kind of pressure that he will face under game conditions. Lay-up shooters should be yelled at, swiped at by defensive hands, and sometimes forced at the last moment to drastically alter their shooting movements in practice because they will be confronted with such during a game. Only in this way, will lay-up shooting done in practice help to improve the quality of performance in the game situation.

Movement Fundamentals (Pivoting, Starting, Running, and Stopping*)

There are innate differences among people, yet it is believed that any basketball player can learn to run reasonably fast and move quickly by utilizing proper movement mechanics. That is, the apparent differences in running and movement abilities of high school and college age players are usually caused as much by faulty employment of mechanics as they are by innate differences. The use of proper mechanics in pivoting, starting, running, and stopping should enable the so-called "slow" boy to improve

*Jumping may also be considered to be a basic movement skill that is quite important in the game of basketball. Full treatment of the mechanical aspects of jumping may be found in the section, "Jumping in Held Ball Situations." The fundamentals presented in that section may be generally considered as proper fundamentals to use in all basketball situations that require jumping ability.

his speed significantly, and will perhaps, cause the so-called "fast" boy to move even faster.

PRINCIPLES OF PERFORMANCE

1. The first step should be long and close to the floor in order to acquire speed quickly.

2. The farther the player runs from the starting position the more upright he should be.

3. Being able to move with quick bursts of speed and controlled speeds is most useful to players in basketball.

4. Running in basketball is usually a compromise between speed and being under control so that the player can stop quickly.

5. Quick movements should involve the use of the principle that the shortest distance between two points is a straight line.

6. Running in a curved path or in cutting by a player is most effectively accomplished if the player accelerates on the curve; if he cuts the radius as short as possible; if he has a fairly wide base; if he has his weight and center of mass toward the inside; and if he leans toward the inside.

7. To stop effectively the center of mass must be first moved to the rear.

8. To maintain balance after stopping the center of mass must be shifted from the rear to a position over the base of support.

9. The faster a player is running, the more he must lower his center of mass in order to stop effectively.

Pivoting is a skill used a great deal in both offensive and defensive basketball. The use of the pivot in the pick and roll pattern has been an effective maneuver for many years, and the use of the defensive pivot to prevent a "backdoor" pass being made is quite common. The stride in the pivot should be fairly long and close to the floor to insure that there is maximum quickness and stability. The first step, after the pivot, should be taken in the direction of the intended path that the player wishes to follow. The front pivot should be used whenever it is mandatory that the player maintain constant eye focus on the ball or on another player. The rear or reverse pivot should be used when quickness of movement is the main objective.

Most players are not as quick as they could be because of the lack of use of proper mechanics in movement. This is an extremely crucial fact because basketball is more often a game of quickness than it is a game of speed. The first step in any forward movement should be long and close to the floor. The player should lean forward in the acceleration phase of the movement. To acquire speed the player should run with a long stride and a high knee lift, and once the initial acceleration phase has ended the player should be running in an upright position. Whenever quickness or speed is the objective, the player should pick the shortest distance between the starting point and the desired objective as the desired path to travel. This means running in a straight line if no obstacles are in the way. Such running is executed so that the player runs a path that involves two connected straight lines as the cut is made around another player. (See drawing below.)

Basketball is a game where full speed is seldom achieved by a player and very infrequently warranted. The basketball player must always be ready to stop and change direction quickly, and this suggests that a compromise must be reached between the use of outright speed and the use of controlled speed so that he can drop quickly or change direction in a hurry. A basketball player is most effective when he can start quickly and move with "controlled speed" to a given spot on the floor.

The faster a player is moving, the more difficult it is to stop quickly and to change direction. If a player is moving very fast at the moment he desires to stop, then his center of mass will have to be lowered considerably for this to be effective. The center of mass should be lowered and allowed to shift to the rear of the base of support in such a situation. If the player can touch another object, he can decrease his momentum considerably faster than he can do so on his own. It may be advantageous for a player to touch another player or to contact the floor with his hands in order to stop quickly. Once the stopping movement has taken place, the center of mass will once again have to be shifted back over the base of support or the player will lose his balance and fall. The player may utilize either the stride foot stance position or the parallel foot stance in stopping. The stride foot stop seems to be the most effective one to use because the base of support is widened in the direction in which balance is needed, that is in the rear-forward direction rather than in the sideward direction.

Many players do not take advantage of the great opportunity afforded them for freeing a cut around another player. If the player will accelerate on the cut or curve and utilize proper mechanics, centripetal force will aid

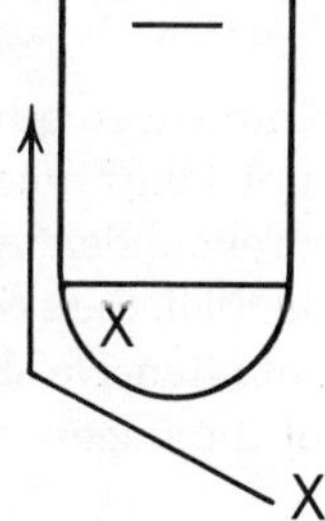

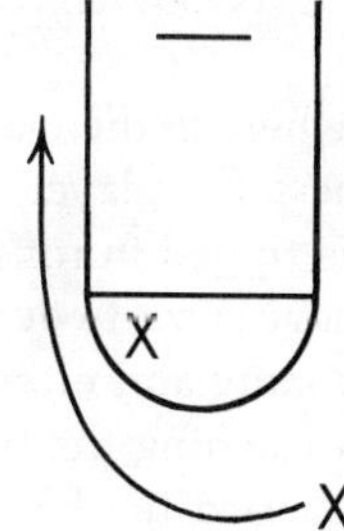

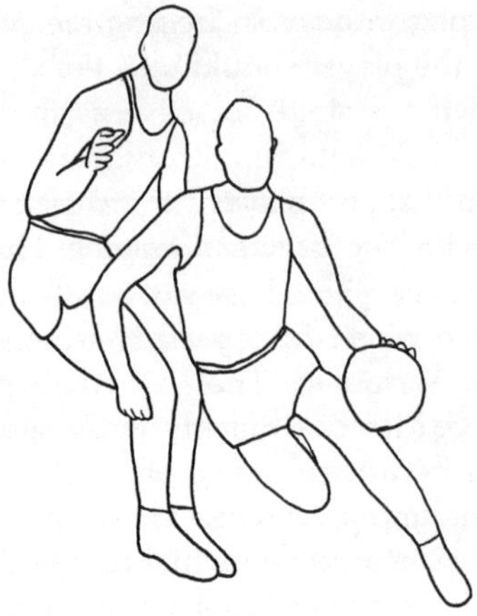

Accelerating on the cut.

him in breaking loose from his opponent. In such action the radius of the cut should be made as short as possible. The player should lean toward the inside of the curve and allow his weight and center of mass to move in that same direction. He should also have a fairly wide base of support as he makes the cutting movement. This will insure him that he will have proper balance as he moves. Whenever a cut is made, it should be made in the form of two subsequently connected straight lines rather than in a curved path. Many opportunities to score are lost merely because a cutter has not taken the shortest path that is available as he cuts around a screen set by a teammate or by a post man.

It must be stated that in most instances skill development in these areas has been sadly neglected. A mediocre player may be changed into a competent one by having him make proper use of quickness. His offensive and defensive ability in basketball could be greatly improved as a result.

Offensive Rebounding (Tipping In)

Perhaps nowhere in the world of sports is disappointment so quickly turned into happiness for player, coach, and fan alike as when a missed shot in basketball is tipped in for a score by an offensive rebounder. As taller and taller men have come to dominate the game of basketball, the skill of tipping has become more and more evident as an important offensive skill. Tipping is the act of catching the ball on the inner sides of the finger tips and then pushing it toward the basket.

Some principles of performance in tipping are presented here.

PRINCIPLES OF PERFORMANCE

1. A player can reach approximately 6 inches higher with the use of one hand rather than with two hands in tipping. However, some coaches believe that beginning players should use two hands when learning this skill.
2. In every instance a correct tip is a catch no matter how momentarily the ball is held.
3. The ball is tipped with the fingers, while the thumb may help to balance the ball on rare occasions.
4. The ball should be tipped with the arm held at full elbow estension. The arm, if at all possible, should never be brought down toward the floor as the ball is caught.
5. Eye contact with the ball should be maintained at all times.
6. The ball should be caught as close to the basket as possible.
7. The tip is executed by finger flexion. Some wrist flexion is used but not very much.
8. Timing the jump so as to catch the ball at the correct spot is the key to successful tipping.

The skill of tipping can be executed with the use of one hand or with two hands. But there is much evidence to suggest that one hand tipping is the far superior method to use in most situations. However, there are times when two hand tipping is the best. The largest single advantage that one hand has over two hand tipping is that a player can reach approximately 6 inches higher with one hand than he can reach with two hands. If the tipper will reach with one hand and move his opposite arm down along side his body depressing one shoulder, he elevates the other shoulder. The anatomy of the shoulder is such that the humerus swings from a movable base so the now elevated shoulder will allow for more efficient and lengthened reach upward being made by the hand. Coaches often suggest that novices should master the two hand tipping skill and then switch to the one when they have achieved a certain skill level in the game of basketball. This concept is subject to questioning because it may well be that two hand tipping is a distinct skill from one hand tipping in that different muscle patterns are used. If this is true, then learning the two hand tip will have little transfer to the learning of the one hand skill of tipping. Young players would be better off starting in immediately with learning how to tip with one hand and two hands as if they are separate skills.

The tip is always a catch, no matter how momentary that catch might be. It is true that the ball can be slapped into the basket, but the successful slap tip is almost always pure luck, and coaches and teachers are concerned

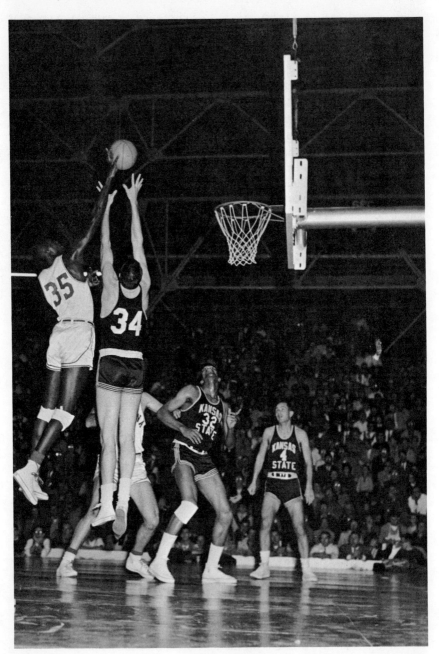

The catch in the one-hand tip-in.

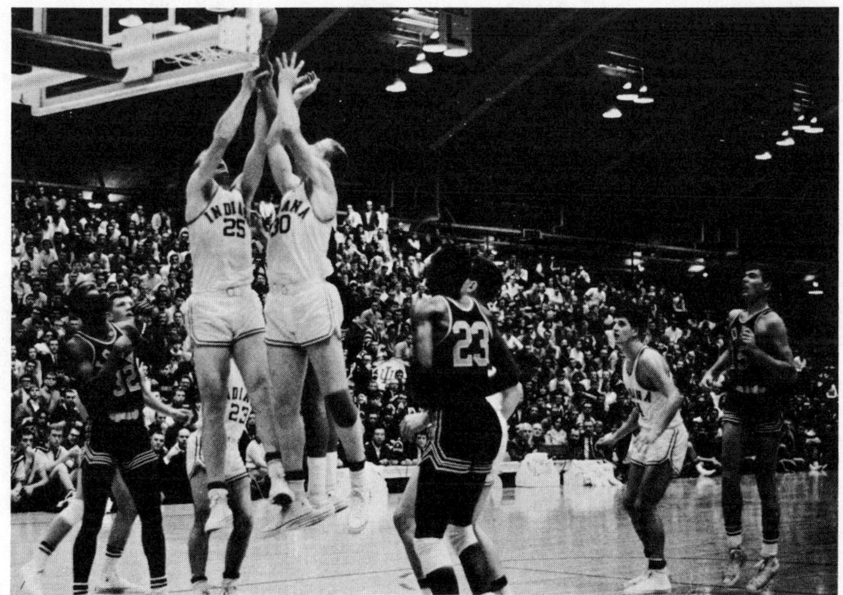

Tipper in full extension.

with the use of skills in which chance does not play such an important role. The tip is executed by hyperextension of the fingers in the momentary catching phase and flexion of the fingers in the "shooting" phase. The thumb may act to balance the ball throughout the tip, but the work of the tip is done by the fingers. Good tippers avoid using the wrist to a great extent in the execution of the tip except in a situation where the ball is caught some distance from the basket. In a case where the distance is over 6 feet from the basket there is always a question as to whether a rebound taken that far away should be tipped or caught firmly and brought down to the floor by the player. In any case, the elbow should be fully extended during the entire tipping motion. None of the impetus for the tip should come from any flexion-extension movement at the elbow joint. Beginners often make the mistake of bringing the ball down by flexing the elbow joint. This is a serious mistake. The ball should not be brought down unless absolutely necessary, and if it must be brought down before the tip is made, it should be brought down with the tip of the elbow held high. Also, if the rebounder will utilize proper one hand jump shooting procedures and keep his elbow fully extended, then he will contact the ball as close to the basket as possible. This is, of course, a great advantage because the accuracy of the tipping action drops off very quickly as the distance from the basket increases.

In order to be able to execute a good tip in, the rebounder must move into the most advantageous position as quickly as possible. Also he must time his jump so that he reaches the ball in the desired position at the apex of his jump. To accomplish this the rebounder must act quickly and aggressively. As the shot is taken, or as a shot is anticipated, the potential tipper must be in motion. He must keep his eyes on the ball all the time that he is in motion in an attempt to get into a good position. He must take a reading on the ball as it is in flight and attempt to determine its ultimate destination. He asks himself the following questions. Will it be short, long, to the right, or to the left? Once he decides on the answer he must move quickly. He must get to the closest position near the basket that he considers to be advantageous for rebounding the shot. Just as is done in defensive rebounding, the tipper must be careful not to get too far underneath the basket or the ball will bounce out beyond him and he will lose the chance to tip the ball into the basket.

While keeping his eyes on the ball at all times, the tipper secures his position and gathers himself in preparation for jumping for the ball. He lowers his center of mass in order to be able to jump high. The tipper must next anticipate the bounce of the ball off the rim or board and make his jump accordingly. He should avoid bouncing up and down in anticipation of the rebound of the ball. If the ball hangs on the rim momentarily or takes a high bounce off the rim or board, the tipper should shuffle his feet and move to a new advantageous position if necessary but remain gathered for the jump.

Defensive rebounders will attempt to block and screen out the tipper, and the tipper must attempt to counter this move. The first thing that the tipper must do is to keep his eyes on the ball. Thus he can only sense by his peripheral vision where the defensive rebounder is located. (He may take his eyes off the ball momentarily, but in doing so he runs the risk of losing its pattern of flight and rebound.) However, quick movements made by the tipper often enable him to move by the blocker. If the defensive rebounder turns his back on the tipper too quickly, the tipper should have no problem moving around him and getting into a good offensive position near the basket to attempt a tip. If contact is made with the defensive rebounder, this will reduce in half the momentum of the charging offensive rebounder. For this reason contact should be avoided. If it cannot be avoided, the tipper must make a new start in an attempt to get by the blocking defensive rebounder. Feints and rolls are often successfully used in moving around the defensive blocker. Kinesthetic and tactual information can be utilized to a great extent in this attempt to avoid the blocker, thus freeing the eyes to follow the flight of the ball.

Defensive Rebounding

Rebounding is the act of retrieving an opponent's missed shot as the ball reflects off the goal or basket. The act of catching the ball as it falls short of the basket, board, or the rim is also considered a part of this action. While this definition limits the discussion to that of defensive rebounding, many of the techniques and principles used in this skill are also applicable to offensive rebounding other than the act of tipping the ball into the basket. (See page 68.)

PRINCIPLES OF PERFORMANCE

1. The ball should be caught, as it is rebounded, with as much vigor as possible, even to the extent that the slap of the hands against the ball is often clearly audible.
2. The ball should usually be caught with the arms fully extended.
3. When possible the ball is retrieved slightly in front of the body rather than directly above it.
4. The spread eagle technique of rebounding, wherein the arms and legs are extended in front of the body, is considered the most effective method to use.
5. The rebounder wishing to initiate a fast break after he catches the ball must lead with his head turned in the direction of the anticipated throw as he returns to the floor.

There are three primary methods employed by a team in effectively rebounding the ball. The first method requires little explanation since it involves just having the rebounders immediately "crash" to their separate rebounding positions close to the basket as the ball is shot at it. The objective of the team in using this method is to secure for themselves as quickly as possible the two, three or more inside rebounding positions. It should be noted that the inside rebounding positions are not directly underneath the basket but rather 2 to 5 feet distance away from it. Too many young and inexperienced rebounders move rapidly to their stations, but end up being almost directly underneath the basket. Often then they helplessly watch the ball bounce off the rim or backboard and go over their heads into the waiting hands of an offensive rebounder.

A second method involves an entirely different concept of rebounding than the one described above. The crash method can be characterized as a "let's go get it" method and its successful use is dependent upon the players being very aggressive. Whereas the second method can be termed a "they can't get the ball if they are kept behind us" method. It is more

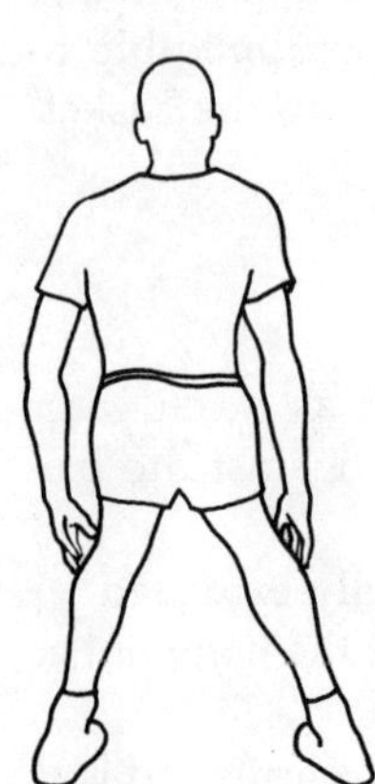

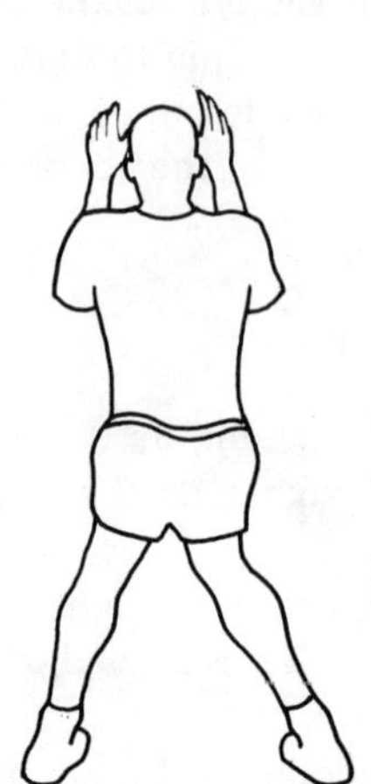

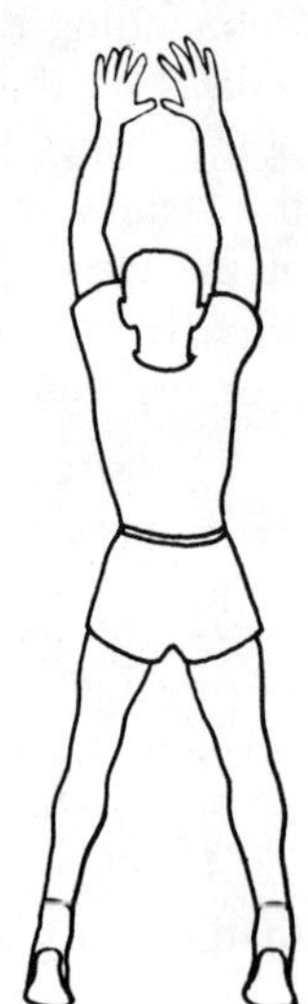

Jumping in a tipping action.

defensive in concept. This method involves the screening out of the offense from the boards. To illustrate, when a shot is taken at the basket, the defensive player retreats quickly a few steps, while at the same time watching his assigned men very closely. When the offensive player makes a move to rebound the ball, the defensive player pivots and cuts him off by stepping into his path. This keeps him from going toward the basket. He does not immediately attempt to retrieve the ball. If the offensive player moves to the inside of the defensive player, he makes a rear reverse pivot and takes one additional step to cut him off from going toward the basket. If the offensive player moves to the outside of him, a front pivot is utilized to accomplish the cut off. The front pivot is also used if both the players find themselves close to the basket because this will narrow the range of movement that the offensive player has at his disposal in his attempt to elude the defensive man. The ultimate team goal when using this particular rebounding method is to have all five offensive players screen out from the basket so effectively that the missed shot could actually fall to the floor before it is retrieved by the defensive rebounder. Many coaches like to use this method of rebounding because it enables them to fix responsibility for rebounding effectively on definite players.

A third method often used is a compromise between the crash and screening out methods. It is probably the method most commonly used by

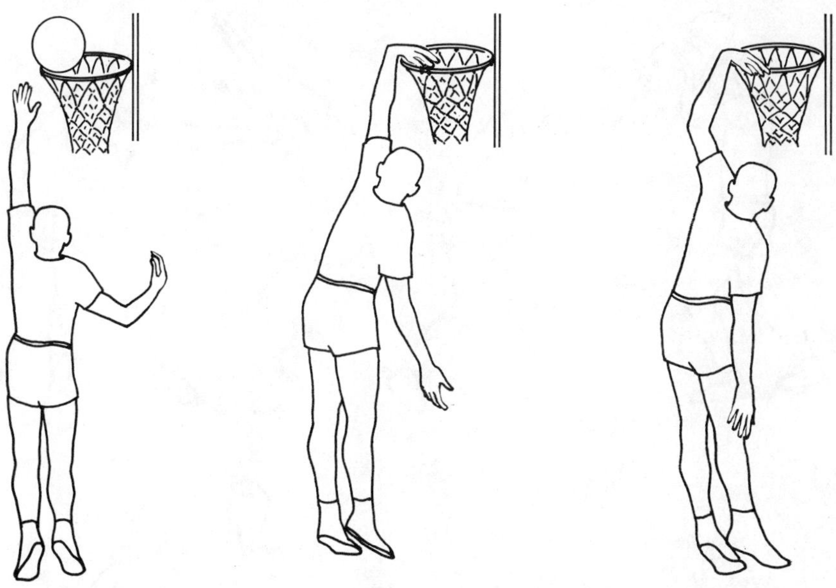

teams today in basketball. In this method the defensive player retreats and cuts off the potential rebounder with the use of almost the same techniques as discussed under the screening out method. The difference is that once body contact has been momentarily established at the cut-off position, the defensive rebounder then turns and goes immediately after the ball. The concept embodied in the use of this method is to momentarily attempt to halt the momentum of the offensive rebounder and then to crash toward the board for the ball. This method is particularly successful when used by forwards. Coaches might want their guards to use the screening out method, their forwards the combination method, and let their big center use the crash method in going for the ball as it rebounds off the backboard.

Regardless of the rebound method used by a team the final act of securing the ball in the hands is the same for all methods. The ball should be rebounded with as much vigor as possible. The rebounder should aggressively grasp the ball even to the extent that an audible slap by his hands can be heard. Furthermore, the ball should be caught with the arms fully extended. This makes the rebounder measure as tall as possible in reach height. It also enables him to secure possession of the ball at the earliest possible time. The most successful rebounders extend their arms between a 45 and a 60 degree angle from the transverse plane rather than extending their arms directly over their heads as they catch the ball. This, of course,

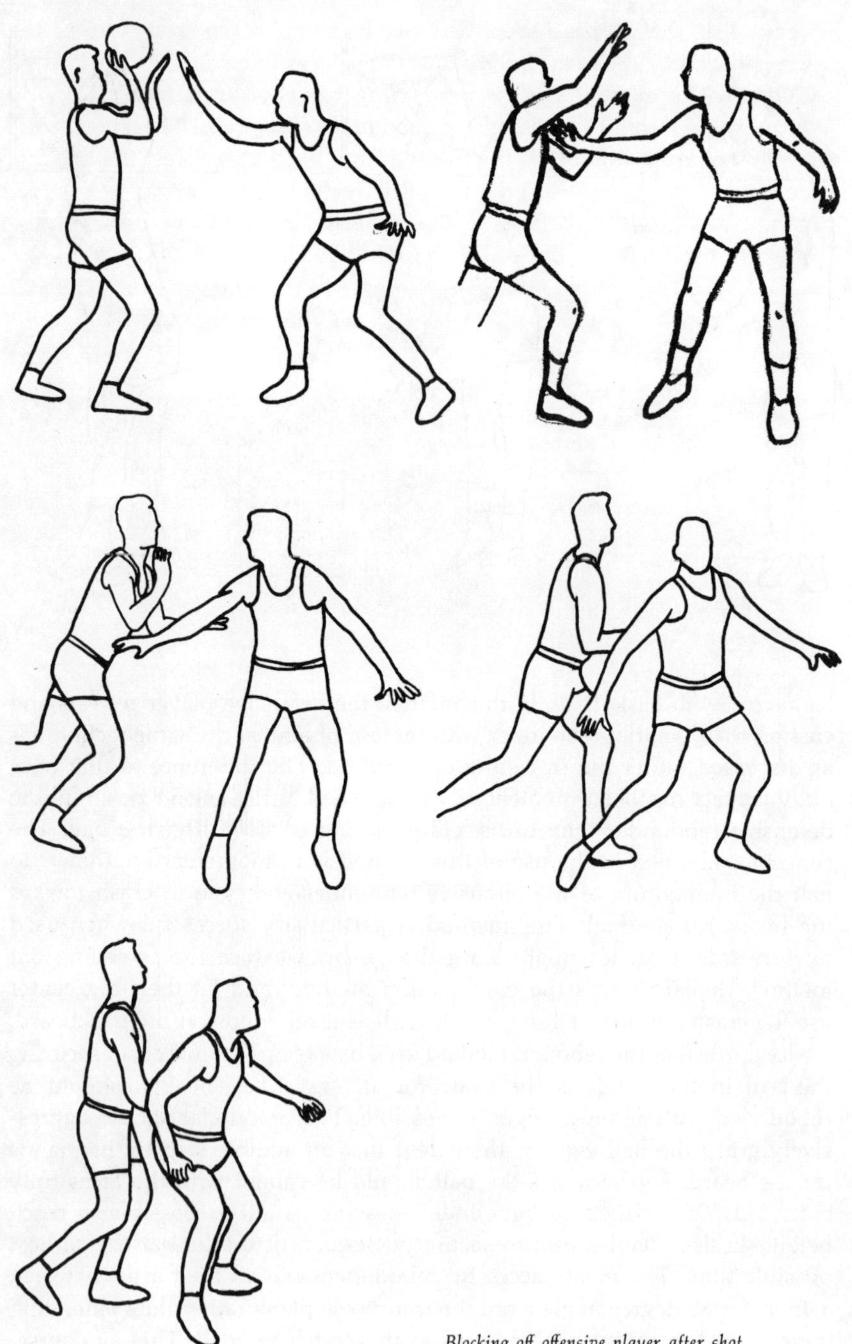

Blocking off offensive player after shot.

means that the ball is rebounded out in front of the body rather than perpendicularly above the body. Thus the ball is protected from the grasping hand of an opponent who is attempting to rebound it from a position immediately behind the defensive rebounder's position. The spread eagle position of arms and legs is the best position to use to protect the ball from the opponent. The arms and legs in this position are thrown out in front of the body and spread apart. As the ball is caught it may be brought down and into the body by flexion of the elbows. Often it is best to keep the ball as high as possible after rebounding it. With the legs and elbows in this position the opponents have a difficult time getting close enough to harass the rebounder with much success.

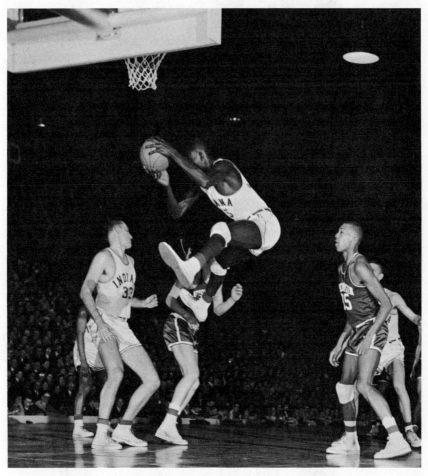

The spread eagle position in rebounding.

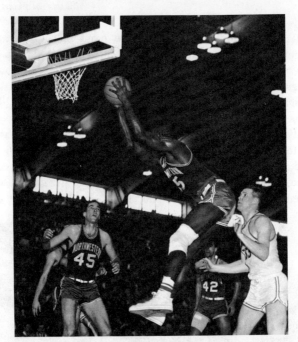

Holding the ball high on the rebound.

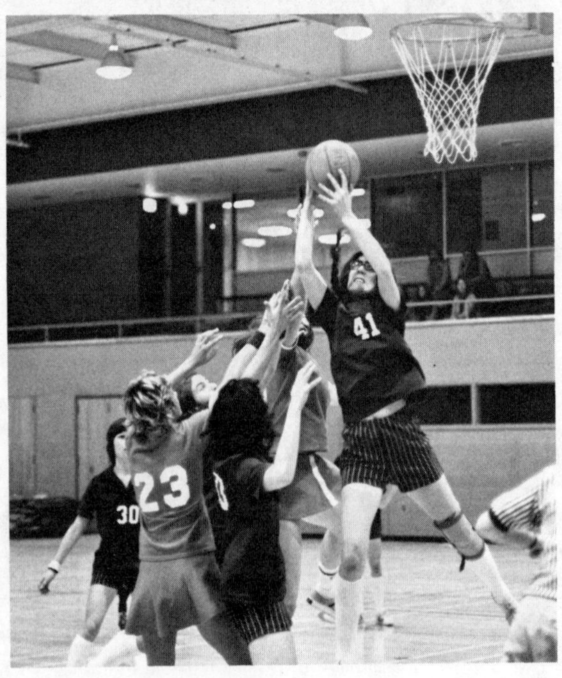

Defensive player legally following the flight of the ball. (Photograph courtesy of Barbara Anderson.)

If at all possible the ball should be caught, but sometimes the rebounder can only get close enough to the ball to bat it with one hand to a teammate. Therefore, the rebounder should have some general idea where his teammates are at all times. If he knows where they are, he should not be afraid to slap the ball vigorously to a teammate. If the team's offensive plans call for the use of the fast break, the rebounder has the added responsibility of attempting to initiate the fast break with an outlet pass being made to a teammate. This can be done effectively only if the rebounder leads with his turned head as he comes to the floor after securing the ball. If on the other hand, the rebounder waits until he is down to the floor to turn and look for the outlet man then precious time has been wasted and the fast break possibility is lost. This move by the defender is done by merely turning the head and looking as he is coming down with the ball. Thus, the outlet pass can be executed immediately when the rebounder returns to the floor. The highly skilled rebounder has had also to master the skill of throwing the outlet pass while he is still in the air. This is an extremely difficult skill to perform, but it is the quickest way known to have a team get a fast break under way.

One final point involves a good example of how a rule change can motivate players to create a new technique and it is found in the skill of rebounding. A few years ago, a rule was adopted that stated that it was a foul for a successful rebounder with the ball to move it back and forth across the front of his chest when the elbows were pointing outward. This had been a favorite technique that rebounders had used to prevent defensive players from slapping at the ball and dislodging it from their grasp. The rule was created because it was believed that this "elbow swinging" technique was unnecessarily rough and created situations in which injuries might occur. The question for the rebounder then became, how to protect the ball from the hands of the defenders without fouling them. A technique was then developed that is gaining wide acceptance by many rebounders. The rebounder in using it just wraps his arms around the ball and bends at the waist so that his torso and his arms cover the ball. With the ball protected in this manner, it becomes virtually impossible for a defender to dislodge the ball from the rebounder without fouling him.

Foul Shooting

By 1902 the rules governing the awarding of a foul toss for personal infractions of the rules to certain selected personnel (and even many of the technical infractions of all the rules) were established as they relate to the distance of the attempt and the value of the successful free toss (except

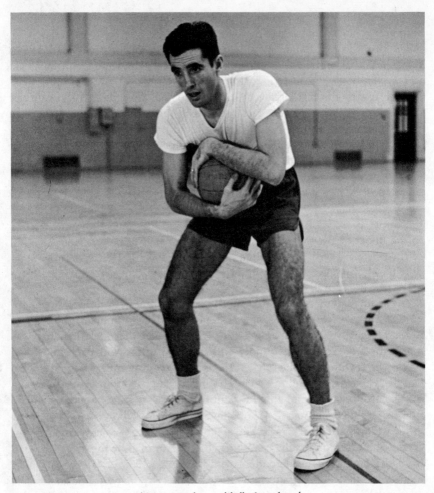

Arms wrapped around ball after rebound.

for minor changes). They have remained in effect up to the present day. The free throw then as now must be attempted unhindered, and is executed from a distance of 15 feet from the basket. The distance was 20 feet in only one year, 1905–1906.

Up to 1923 one player was designated as the shooter and attempted all the tosses for his team. The idea being that "the value of a foul would depend on the skill of the team at throwing goals. Accordingly, some member of the team was designated to make the free throw."*

*Naismith, James: *Basketball,* Association Press, New York, 1941, P. 71.

Such designated players became so proficient that it was almost an automatic point when they made a toss. Anderson of Lafayette College holds the all time college record of 764 successful free throws made out of 930 attempts, an .822 average over four years, 1915–19. It was not unusual for the single tosser for each team to make from 12 to 15 successful tosses out of possible 15. Most of the tossers were perfectionists who spent a large portion of the practice period shooting free tosses.

There are many styles of shooting foul shots that might be used including the one-hand push, two-hand underhand toss, two-handed push, overhead one and two-hand push, and the jump shot.

It appears from the meager research available that there will be greater success attainable from the underhand two-hand toss than from the other styles for most players. However, most of the research studies used subjects who had varying years of training and all had had experience with certain styles before being tested, which would affect the validity of the experiments. Also, since foul shooting involves the element of chance, many trials would have to be accomplished before the reliability could be established.

Several modern day top performers such as Bill Sharman of the University of Southern California (who made 19 free tosses out of possible 19 in conference play one year and also led the professional N.B.A. basketball league in the highest successful percentage in foul tossing in 1953–54 as a member of the Boston Celtics) and Tony Lavelli of Yale (who held the modern national college record for a four-year period having a .781 average) were one-handed shooters. Also, many good foul shooters have used the two-handed push shot. The main argument in favor of using the one push shot has been that the player will be more proficient if he uses the same style of shooting from the free throw lane that he uses from the field. Also since the underhand style of shooting from the field is no longer used, much practice time would have to be spent on learning a new shot to be used only a few times each game.

On the other hand, it is the opinion of some coaches and teachers that for most players the under-hand shot might be the most proficient. The reasons for the underhand shot being considered the best for most players is that it is one of the few "natural" shots in basketball. Most beginners can execute it with a reasonable degree of accuracy. It takes less strength for its execution as evidenced by young children's ability to throw farther with this motion than with any other with the exception of the one-hand baseball throw. Therefore, it is reasoned then it will be easier to execute when a player is fatigued. Also, it should be more accurate because both hands would work together longer in executing the shot and the hands are on the ball longer (a total length of time) than with most other foul shooting styles.

Yet, it is argued that the successful one-handed shooter might have been more successful if he had spent the same time and effort on the underhand shot and therefore had confidence in his ability to execute it. However, the one-hand shooter may be just as relaxed and as sound a shooter using his style as in using underhand method. Taking into consideration all the arguments presented here both pro and con it is believed that most players will continue to use the one-hand style in foul shooting in the foreseeable future.

Regardless of the style of shooting used it is believed that certain common principles of performance can be established that will apply to any style. These principles are enumerated below as they apply to the one-hand style of shooting. With only the elimination of those items that obviously do not apply to other styles and with some modification of foot and arm positions, the same procedures that are mentioned here may be used by most players in spite of their preferred style of shooting. The one-handed foul shot is executed the same as the one-handed shot from the field and a detailed analysis of this shot is included in the section on shooting.

PRINCIPLES OF PERFORMANCE

1. The player should dry off the fingertips.

   a. The ball is loosely placed in the hands to establish the sense of feel and either the ball is shaken with the hands by moving the wrist or it is bounced on the floor once or twice. Such movements release tension.

   b. The position of teammates is observed to see if all players are off the foul lines.

2. The feet are placed in a stride position close to the foul line, the right foot in advance of the left (right hand shooter). The toes of the right foot should be pointing inward and the toes of the left slightly outward. The head is kept down to observe correct foot placement; the ball is kept just over head or close to waist to avoid creating tension in the arms.

   a. The ball is moved so that the same grip is used as is used in one hand set shooting. (see pages 51–53.) The ball rests on the fingers, not in the palm of the hand.

3. The player now takes a deep breath. This helps relax the shooter and also prevents the chest area from moving while shooting, which would interfere with accuracy.

4. He looks up at the goal, and focuses his attention on shooting just over the rim (a target point must be selected). The head is held up, and the back kept straight.

5. The knees are slightly bent, the ball is brought back and down, the wrists are flexed, and then the ball is released. If over 1.5 seconds is spent

in this position, the player becomes tense and his accuracy is affected. The wrist and finger action is executed as the ball is released and then the follow-through is done rhythmically.

a. The arms and the body follow through are pointed directly in line with the basket.

6. The ball should be released with a slight backspin which will make it easier to catch on the rebound and may cause it to go into the basket from off the board or back rim. It has been estimated that a correctly delivered shot will make three revolutions before reaching the goal.

7. The ball must be tossed softly in harmony with the rhythm of the entire body.

8. The eyes should not follow the ball in flight, but should be fixed on the target. However, if a player can concentrate on the target until after the ball is released from the hands, the accuracy of the shot is not affected if he follows it afterwards with his eyes in flight.

9. The shooter should be sure not to step toward the basket too soon. This can be prevented by keeping at least one foot firmly on the floor until the shot has been made or missed.

10. The least amount of extraneous movements possible made by the shooter aids in the accuracy of the shot. A rhythmic, smooth movement assures that a soft, accurate shot is accomplished.

Practicing foul shots should be done in such a manner that they are performed as they would be in a game. The same idea should be used in the physical education classes as far as it is practicable. Play should be stopped at intervals and the whole group (physical education class or varsity squad) should be asked to shoot 25 shots in a series of one or two with the other players usually lined up in their proper position along the foul lines. Occasionally the players should shoot without anyone being along the foul lines to stimulate technical foul situations. Careful shooting should be insisted upon as improper practice will become habitual and be used during competition. Horseplay permitted during the shooting of foul shots is usually uncalled for under most conditions.

Screening

Screening is the offensive act of placing one's body in the path of a defensive player so as to impede his progress. Thus, it is most often used by one player to momentarily free a teammate so he can attempt a shot, make a cut toward the basket, and/or receive a pass. Screening has long been used as an important part of offensive basketball. The so-called "Eastern" United States basketball teams were for many years characterized by the screening techniques used by their offensive players.

PRINCIPLES OF PERFORMANCE

1. The screener should spread his legs so he makes a wide base with them. He must set the screen one normal step from the player to be screened.

2. The facing screen is the most adaptable one because the screener can adjust so that he can move more readily to a position in the path of the defensive player.

3. The screen from the rear is usually the most effective one to use against some players.

4. The screener should maintain his screening position until momentary contact has been established with the defensive player and then he should move rapidly toward the basket.

5. The screener must be directly in the path of the defensive player and not to one side. Also he must not be moving at the moment of contact.

The purpose of using a screen is to prevent a defensive player from moving to a position where he can continue to effectively guard an offensive player. Originally, screening was done with one player remaining stationary throughout the action and the other player using his teammate, who was in a stationary position, as the screen for the purpose of freeing him so he could cut toward the basket unguarded. The idea for using the stationary screens came from the use that was made of the posts supporting the balconies and ceilings in the old gymnasiums. Players often used these posts to aid them in eluding their defensive opponents much as football ends today use the goal posts to free themselves momentarily from the defensive halfbacks.

Currently, stationary screen techniques are not widely used, but a great variety of other types of screens have been developed to become important parts of most offensive patterns. Many coaches prefer to have their players use the facing screen wherein the screener moves into the path of a defensive player while he is facing directly toward him. This enables the screener to watch the defensive player at all times and to adjust his screening position to the directional path of the defensive player. Another type of screen quite different to the one just mentioned is where the screener turns his back toward the defensive player he is attempting to screen. Upon contact with the defensive player he is in a good position to move toward the basket. Regardless of which method is used the screener should spread his legs so as to form a wide base thus making his body as wide as possible without getting himself into an awkward position. The screener should maintain his position until momentary contact has been made with the defender being screened, or until such time as it is clear that the defender has changed his path of motion to avoid being screened. In either case, maintaining the screening position too long lessens the offensive effectiveness that should result from the screen. Undoubtedly, the screener should move quickly toward the basket in preparation for the possibility of receiving a return pass from his offensive teammate for whom he has just set the screen. If a switch in defensive men has occurred due to the results of the screen, the screener by moving toward the basket quickly can cause the defender he has just screened to be behind him. It is for this reason that screeners are cautioned not to maintain the screen for too long a time.

The description contained in the preceding pages has been that of the old "pick and roll" procedure that played such an important role in the early development of offensive basketball. However, it should be pointed out that only a true *pick* and *roll* situation exists if a facing type screen is used. This is because with the use of facing type screen the screener must utilize a reverse pivot to "roll" toward the basket. It is this movement that gives this offensive maneuver its name. If a back screen is used, the screener merely has to move directly toward the basket after the screen is made. The advantages of the use of each then become immediately obvious. The use of the facing screen enables the screener to execute his screen better because he can see his target longer. He makes last second adjustments so that the defender is more apt to come into contact with him. On the other hand, the use of the back screen, while it is a less effective screen, does enable the screener to move toward the basket more quickly and thus become an offensive threat sooner.

Perhaps the most difficult screen to avoid is the rear screen where the screener approaches the defensive player from the rear. Although the screener must allow enough room for the defender to turn around, it is still very effective and has an element of surprise to it. Its use helps draw many fouls for the screener. This screen is often used by a forward or a pivot man on a defensive guard.

The use of double screens and two man screens are also very effective. The double screen is usually set by two teammates neither of whom has the ball and the object is to attempt to free one of the players so that he may try to make a short jump shot or a cut toward the basket. The double screen is really two single screens set one right after the other. The first screen is set by B. A cut off the screen and immediately peels back to set a screen for B (See drawing). Its use is, naturally, confusing to the defenders

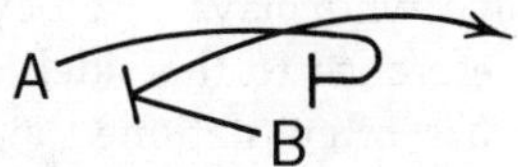

and is especially frustrating to players on teams who like to switch on defense. Two man screens are also effective to use especially in creating mismatches in size or ability by forcing switches to be made by the defensive team. The two man screen is executed by having two screens set instead of one, thus greatly eliminating the possibility of the defensive player eluding the screen by slipping over it or behind it. This is true because the distance the defensive player would have to move to beat the screen is virtually doubled (See drawing).

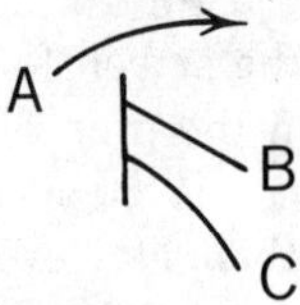

The most recent type of screen being used is called a running screen (which it technically is not or it would be illegal). The screening player runs and then hesitates briefly and then continues on his run . He stops just long enough to let a teammate execute a quick shot at the basket. This type of screening takes excellent timing.

The practice time allotted to screening procedures should be in proportion to the importance they play in the offense selected by the coach. Most coaches feel that screening is a basic part of the game of basketball and it should be given the same attention by the players in practice as dribbling, passing, and one-on-one offensive and defensive procedures.

Playing the Post

A player who can perform well in a post or around the key position is always in demand by the coach and players. The coach can easily build an offense around a good post man, probably easiest of all players. The good players rely on such a player to provide offensive impetus.

There is no difference in the pivot and post positions. In basketball parlance the terms are often used interchangeably. Basically, the low post player is one who is a scoring threat at all times. On the other hand, the high post player may be only a feeder and passer and not primarily an offensive threat. The position of the players (high or low post) on the court may also influence the determination of the definition that is applied to these terms. A player on offensive who plays just beyond the foul line in the middle of the court with reference to the sideline is thought of as a *high* post. Double post players are often stationed at the end of the foul line toward the center of the court and just at the beginning of the foul circle. A low post player is one who is usually stationed near the basket. However, basically the general all around play is the same for the low and high post player.

There are many moves used to make post play successful. Some of these moves depend upon the location of the opposition, the body build and skill of the performer and the score and period in the game. The information outlined below includes the main steps to follow playing such positions in most situations.

PRINCIPLES OF PERFORMANCE

1. A target is set with the hands by the post player so that the passer knows where to throw the ball when he is ready to release it.

2. The ball is received high at an elevation even with the chest or even higher, if players are converging and double teaming on the post player. The overhead two-handed pass is one of the best to use in passing to a big post man because it can be caught above and away from the defense. Also if he catches the ball in a shooting or passing position, it means that there is less chance of an interception taking place or that the player will be tied up with the ball.

A post player often roams back and forth near the front of the basket and from the foul circle to directly beneath the basket. It is possible to have a post player stationed much farther away from the basket and in front or toward either sideline. If the player in this position is a continuous offensive threat, that is, shooting often, then that player is classified as playing a post position.

Normally, the low post man should not call for a pass to be thrown to him from the guards (when they are far out on the floor and well defensed) when he is in a deep position near the basket because the chances for an interception taking place are usually great. When the post player has taken a position out beyond the foul line, he becomes a high post player and passes to him are less apt to be intercepted. Usually passes are more effective to the post delivered from the side players than from the players stationed directly in front of him when the team is playing against a loose man-to-man defense. However, a clever passer who keeps the defense guessing at all times can pass to the post effectively from in the front position.

3. When the ball is caught, it should be protected with the body and elbows. The ball may be caught with the palms of the hands close together and facing each other and in a horizontal position, one above the other, if the defensive man continuously slaps at the ball as the post player is catching it.

4. The ball should be turned from side to side by rolling the wrist. This movement provides added protection against the slapper.

5. The low post including the hook shot player must be able to turn and shoot with either hand and from either side of the basket. If the post

is not able to shoot with either hand, a two-handed shot from the non-preferred side may be used.

The low post player should have one or two favorite shots he likes to use, but he should be able to execute a shot from his left and right side (one of the shots from one side may be a two- or one-handed turn or jump shot), composed of a jump shot, a hook shot and once in awhile a fade shot. High school post men should be able to use at least two of the above shots to be effective unless they are extremely tall. Shots such as the turn and underhand flip should add to the variety of shots available and may make a post player more effective.

6. The post player should secure good floor position, which is usually 4 or 5 feet from the basket and near the foul lane. This is done so as to be as close to the basket as possible and still have room to move laterally in order to execute an effective shot. He should always try to stay in the line of deployment. In other words, he should always try to maintain a straight line between the ball, himself, and the basket. This makes it very difficult for the defensive man to decide which side of him to place himself on defense.

7. The player should move quickly to the desired spot at which he wants to receive the pass so the defense cannot crowd him out too far on the court. Patience is the key word the post player must remember when he tries to catch the ball in an advantageous shooting or passing (feeding) position.

8. He must be able to move and know where the lines and marking on the courts are in relation to the basket and playing court. Some coaches draw special lines on the court for early season practice to help the players learn the court locations.

9. Many teams have the post player give a signal when the ball will be passed in to him by means of his location on the court. For example, he may raise his hand or hands, and move to a high post position which is a signal that he wants the ball thrown to him; make a head and/or shoulder movement indicating the ball is to be passed into him, regardless of his location.

The post player must come to meet the passed ball rather than remain stationary unless he is already moving toward the basket or is in a position out deep on the court. Just one step is often all he needs to take to get free to receive the ball. A bounce pass may be made to the post player when he is stationed far out on the court beyond the foul line. The post player will then be able to turn and drive toward the basket with the ball.

10. The ball should be hidden from the opposing defensive man at all times. This is done by attempting to place the body between the ball and the defensive man. This also involves being able to hand off properly to

cutting players without the defensive man being able to hand off properly to cutting players without the defensive man being able to see who has the ball. A heavy and broad post player is usually always a better target to throw to than a tall thin pivot man. However, the thin post player, who can cut to the proper position rapidly with or without the use of a screen from a teammate, may in the end make the better post. This may be true when he has the ability to use his elbows legally to increase body width and when he is superior in rebounding and all around maneuverability to the heavy player.

11. A fake is made to draw the opposing defensive man up into the air or in the opposite direction of the intended move. The fakes and feints that a post man uses to free himself so he can receive the ball and shoot it often are determined by his size and the size of the opposition; distance from the basket; the height the ball is received; direction he is moving, etc. However, a quick upward movement of the head or a glance upward with the eyes toward the basket often gives the illusion that a shot is being attempted and a shoulder or knee dip or step out may cause the opposition to move in the desired, but opposite, direction to the intended one. These moves are among the most effective fakes now in use by good post players.

12. The eyes of the defensive player should be focused on the buttocks or middle of the body of the offensive pivot player. This focus is maintained until the pivot has committed himself as to his intentions. He makes his move to screen the offensive post man as he attempts to rebound the ball after a shot is made by his teammates. The offensive post player should not be permitted to move too close to the basket at the time of the rebounding. The defensive man should spread his feet and stay low and turn to screen out the offensive post player when he moves to get the rebound. A spread eagle position with the legs is made (on the jump) and the ball is caught as high as possible. The ball after being caught is usually kept in a high position unless it is necessary to wrap the arms around it.

13. A short person guarding a tall offensive post must stay close to him and often get in front of him to prevent him from receiving the ball. He may also attempt to intercept the passes made to him. A continuous shifting of the guarding position so that the defensive player moves from the side to the rear, to the side to the front of the offensive player, may be necessary.

A tall person guarding a short person usually should stay away from him as much as 2 feet or more when he is fairly close to the basket. Most of the time a position from the rear is satisfactory to use since the tall person can block the short person's shots and he must be far enough away to prevent the short man from driving in for a setup. The tall person may also be able to deflect passes made to a short person from a side guarding position. Occasionally it may be advantageous to even play in front of him. The cleverness of the small post and the maneuverability of the tall guard will determine the position best suited for him to play.

14. In shooting any shot the offensive post should keep two hands on the ball as long as possible. In addition, the shot must be soft enough to enable the offensive players to rebound it. Any fade away shot must be shot with caution since the shooter most likely will not be able to rebound the ball if the shot is missed.

Intercepting Passes

Interception of passes (by players using a man-to-man defense) to an intended receiver is often done rather spasmodically and often without plan. The following ideas are presented with the hope that the coach and players will weigh the calculated risk and then act accordingly. The members of a team using a zone defense are constantly striving to intercept passes and hence are not involved specifically in this discussion. However, some of the principles presented here may be utilized by players using any type of defense.

PRINCIPLES OF PERFORMANCE

1. Usually a defensive player should not try too often to intercept a pass unless the situation calls for desperate measures to be undertaken, or unless the opposition is confused or very weak in the execution of passes.
2. The manner of passing and the speed of the pass should be observed very closely before trying to intercept the ball.
3. An attempt to move for the interception should come just after the passer has committed himself. This would usually be as his arms have almost extended from his body and his hands have slid in behind the ball.
4. The anticipated path of the ball should be determined and then the player should move toward (even away from) the passer and in the direction of the path of the ball in its flight.
5. On a long pass the player has more time to determine the direction and path of the ball and can take more chances. Full-court and cross-court passes are the easiest to intercept.
6. The player should normally play close to an intended receiver, but should overshift enough to one side of him to avoid striking him as he moves for the ball.
7. Careless and fancy passers should be watched very closely. Many opportunities for interceptions will arise when playing against such players.
8. Many players have a habit of executing only one or two specific passes when in stressful situations. Therefore, the defensive players should be prepared to attempt to make interceptions under these circumstances if feasible.
9. The more preliminary movements the passer has to make in order

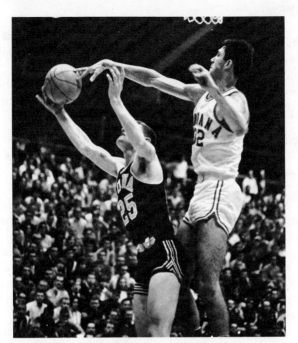

A clean stop by a defensive player.

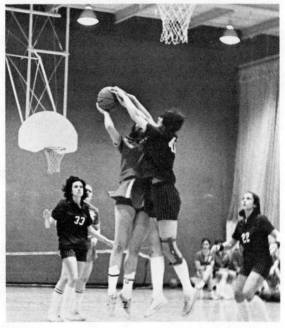

An aggressive defensive player in action. (Photograph courtesy of Judith Zoble.)

to execute the pass (*i.e.* uses arms and body instead of wrist movement only), the more information is given to the would be intercepter on where and how the ball will move when passed.

10. Many players at the last moment telegraph with their eyes where they are throwing the ball. They look at the intended target just as they are ready to release the ball.

11. Forcing a player to change his tempo of passing also opens up opportunities for interceptions to be made. A pressing defense, especially one employed in the backcourt, often creates such situations.

12. Constant changing of stances, foot positions and distances from the opposing offensive players sometimes disconcerts them and also the ones to whom they are passing, thus interceptions can often be made.

13. Occasionally, false moves can be made by the would be intercepter. These false moves may lure the passer into making what he feels is a safe pass, but one which the intercepter will be able to catch easily.

In summary, it might be stated that intercepting passes is an art that, above all, requires patience on the part of the defensive player. It is not usually recommended that players attempt to intercept passes every time the offensive team brings the ball down the floor. Indeed, the "smart" defensive player may under normal circumstances only make two to four attempts each game. The use of any more than this number will alert the offensive player so that he modifies his moves to counteract the attempted stealing action and thus the opportunity to intercept is lessened. The defensive player must wait until he feels the offense is "set up" for an interception. He then must make his move quickly and boldly. Any hesitation at the last moment will probably cause him to miss intercepting the ball, and will likely cause his teammates to have to cover for his "mistake."

Jumping in Held Ball Situations

There are on the average from eight to twelve jump ball situations that occur in college contests and twelve to sixteen such situations happening in high school basketball games. This means that there is a possibility of or at least an opportunity to score a basket or to retain possession of the ball each time a jump is made.

The younger the players, the less advantage height is in a jump. Even with more mature players, timing, coordination and savvy concerning the spot the official will toss the ball are often more important than the height of the jump. Most very tall men fail to mechanically place their legs in the best position for jumping because they have been able most of their playing careers to out jump smaller opponents without having to exert themselves to their maximum jumping capacity.

The principles involved in executing a jump from a stationary position are the same whether it be in the center or foul circle positions. They are as follows:

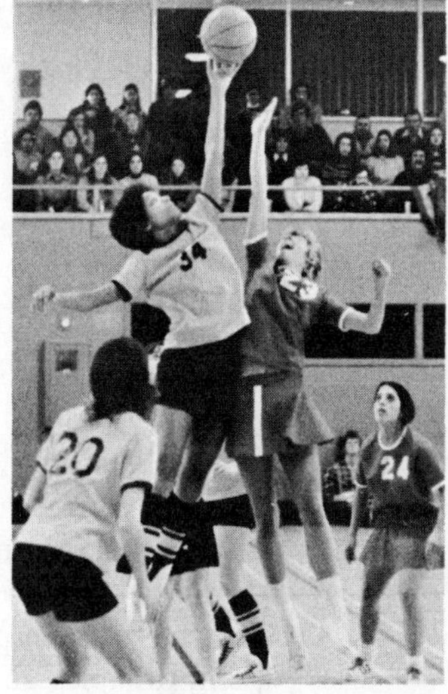

Note full arm reach and torso twist in a jump ball situation. (Photograph courtesy of Barbara Anderson.)

PRINCIPLES OF PERFORMANCE

1. The knees are bowed inward and bent to slightly more than a 45 degree angle.

2. The bottom surfaces of both feet are used to initiate the spring upward. A slight "crowhop" (an extra small hop) may be necessary to help a short, or a poor player, or even a good jumper to jump higher. Just as the official throws up the ball, the center (jumper) moves so both feet touch the circle and jumps upward.

3. The jumper should accent leaving the floor with a final push being made from the big toes.

As the player prepares to tip the ball, his back should be arched so that the tipping arm can be reaching upward to its maximum. The body from the toes to the outstretched arm is extended. The free arm is thrust downward as the jump is made. This increases the reach of the arm used for tipping the ball.

4. Timing the jump so as to tap the ball at the apex of its flight if possible is more important than the ability to jump high. Whereas the tall boy has the advantage in the total height jumped, the shorter player can often start and finish his jump sooner. Normally, the jump should be started just after the ball leaves the official's hand.

5. The position of the feet and the body in preparation for the jump is determined by practice and by the strategy of the situation. However, the jumper should usually place one foot slightly in front of the other foot while facing the circle diameter line from a side or front position. The ball should usually be tapped with the hand closest to the ball in its flight, especially if the opponent is a fine jumper. The right hand is usually used for tapping if the jumper is right handed. The ball can be tapped to the rear easier than to the front if the two jumpers are about equal in ability and jumping height. Also, if a jumper is unable to jump as high as an opponent, his most effective tapping procedure would be to attempt to make a rear tap. It takes more time to turn in the air and tap the ball in any jumping situation.

6. The tipper, if possible, usually catches the ball momentarily with the fingers of the tipping hand. This assures him more control and accuracy in placement of the ball.

7. The ability to use either hand when jumping is an advantage against some opponents, but it usually takes more practice to perfect this movement in order to use either hand equally well at the height of the jump.

Participating in Drills

Participation in drills seems to be an important experience for players to have in a basketball class or on a team. This is especially true for younger players where practice in drills may actually account for over one-half of the class or practice time. While the use of drills seems to be somewhat less important, at least in terms of time spent (as the level of skill increases), it still occupies an integral part of team practice sessions at the college and professional level. Books have been written listing the many types of drills available to the coach or teacher. So, it is not within the scope of this book to attempt to duplicate that effort. It is extremely important, however, that coaches and teachers have some basis for selecting or inventing drills for use by their players. It goes without saying that some drills are better for use than others, and that perhaps the "homemade" drill designed to fit a specific situation is the most valuable. The presentation in this section is an attempt to submit guide lines that may be used in the selection and development of drills.

PRINCIPLES OF DRILL SELECTION AND DEVELOPMENT

1. Drills should contain elements of the crucial actions found in a game situation.

2. Drills should include a crucial point in the execution of a movement.

3. Drills should embody some aspects of the team's offensive and defensive system.

4. Players should normally not participate in a shooting drill alone.

5. Drills should be based on a progressive difficulty scale.

6. Competition can help motivate better performances in drills.

7. Proper team reaction to a specific game situation should be emphasized during the drill activities.

8. As many team players as possible, as often as possible, should be involved in participation in a drill.

9. Drill practice must be purposeful for improvement to take place. Drill participation is helpful only if an attempt is made to recreate the

action found in a game situation. This requires that a certain amount of pressure be present during the action. Taking part in a dribbling drill, for instance, only becomes truly meaningful when some pressure is applied to the dribbler. It is very unrealistic to expect that merely dribbling the ball up and down the length of the floor will help the player to become a better dribbler in the game situation. A transfer of training will only take place if the situations are similar, and it is of little value to a coach to have a dribbler that can perform effectively when he is unmolested only to be ineffective when defensive pressure is applied.

The truly crucial point in the executing of a game movement should be recreated as much as possible in a drill. If, for instance, a coach wants to work on the change of direction dribble, then he should carefully examine, through the use of movies perhaps, the game situation in which a change of direction dribble has often occurred, and then attempt to have his players recreate this situation. All movements should be eliminated from the activity during the drill that are extraneous to the situation.

Drills can also be used to provide a basis for developing proper team reaction to a specific game situation. To illustrate, if a team uses a verbal or body signal to indicate the intended direction that a ball is to be tipped in a jump ball situation, this can be practiced meaningfully by the entire team in a drill situation. The man jumping should never jump without first knowing where he wants to tip the ball and giving a signal to his teammates of his intentions.

Drills should embody a part of a team's offensive or defensive system. This means that many standard drills must be adapted for use so as to fit into the individual team system being used. The use of this adaptation will then be much more meaningful to the players and it will insure that more learning will take place because it more nearly coincides with the conditions found in a game situation. Dribbling drills, for example, can be utilized in such a manner that they involve actions that are part of the team's offensive pattern rather than just line drills. Passing can be used in the situations where passes most often occur in the team's offensive moves (pattern), rather than just passing the ball back and forth across the floor. Adherence to this principle in the use of drills will give the players more practice on developing those skills that they will actually be called upon to perform in the game situation.

It is unusual for a player to have the opportunity to shoot unmolested in a game situation. Even if he is momentarily free there will probably be some opponent rushing at him in an attempt to at least bother him on the shot. For this reason, shooters should almost never be allowed to shoot in practice without some harassment. There is even some evidence to indicate that such shooting may not be real practice of the desired skill at all. Oliphant kept records of daily shooting accomplishments by the varsity and freshman squads at State University of Iowa. He found that there was no significant improvement in prepractice shooting effectiveness throughout the season. The use of shooting drills can be very significant as aids in learning and improving. Yet it also can be virtually a waste of time depending upon the type of drill used during the practice period.

Drills should have an increasing degree of difficulty inherent in their design. It is not easy for the player to maintain interest, and therefore give 100 per cent in effort in participating in a drill that is repetitious and monotonous. Activity in a drill should become increasingly more complex to hold the interest of the player so that his motivational level will remain high. Unchanging and monotonous activity that is not purposeful may preclude that the desired learning will take place.

As many of the players as possible should be involved in the drill activities as often as possible. It is logical to conclude that the more repetitions that are involved in a learning situation, the more likely that the desired learning changes will be reinforced and become habit. Nothing is more detrimental to both effective learning and team conduct than to have long lines of players waiting to take part in a drill situation. Coaches and teachers should develop and/or select drills that will allow for maximum participation by all members of the squad.

Conditioning for Basketball

Often a coach can only do just so much to help improve the level of skill of his players in getting them ready for the playing of the game of basketball. However, there is no excuse that he can offer that is acceptable if his team loses a game that it might have won had the players been in better physical condition. It is believed that he can properly prepare his players relative to the conditioning phase provided he has his players do certain things. Therefore, listed below are general principles that should aid the coach in understanding the nature of the conditioning process and there are also selected principles that he may use as guides in helping him to develop a conditioning program for use by his players. Further information on the conditioning process, since this is only a brief treatise, may be obtained from current physiology of exercise books and research articles found in the bibliography of this book.

PRINCIPLES FOR CONDITIONING FOR BASKETBALL

1. Sustained running is the easiest way to increase general circulo-respiratory fitness. However, in basketball the running pace should be fast, for short distances, and repeated often.

2. Endurance is specific to the given activity under consideration. Basketball players in a game use quick bursts of speed and side-to-side and up-and-back motions. These actions should be a part of their conditioning program.

3. Muscular strength and endurance should be developed in accordance with the need of specific movements (jumping is an example, whereby resistance to it should be offered as the players execute the movement).

4. The use of isometric exercises tend to develop less bulk in the muscle than isotonic exercises, but are functional only for the limb angle in which they are practiced.

5. The use of isotonic exercises, in the long run, tends to produce more favorable results than isometrics.

6. Speed of movement is best developed by the players using many repetitions against a light resistance.

7. To increase strength a muscle must be overloaded. That is, it must be tested against increasing resistance.

8. Players who run long distances will increase general endurance but this will tend to work against the development of speed and quickness.

9. The preseason conditioning program must be quite different from the inseason conditioning program. The needs for these two periods are quite different.

The player in good physical condition is generally thought to have the ability to do sustained work over a long period of time. Thus he is thought to have endurance. Endurance, however, can be conceived of in several different ways. One might speak of general circulo-respiratory endurance as measured by maximum oxygen consumption. One might also speak of endurance as the ability to be able to sustain an effort while performing a specific activity. And, furthermore, one might speak of endurance as the ability to sustain work that is done by a particular muscle group. All of these concepts have meaning for the coach who wants his players to be able to play a full game at full speed and still have enough left at the close of it to put on a press or to stall effectively. In other words, he does not want his players to "run out of gas." Concepts and ideas that may help the coach to achieve his goal of having well-conditioned basketball players are presented here.

Sustained running is the easiest way to increase general circulo-respiratory fitness. Long runs performed at an even pace seem to have no equal in building this type of endurance. The coach may want to encourage his players to participate in this type of activity during the summer months. The coach should stress that staying in shape is a year around job for the dedicated player.

Basketball endurance, however, as is true for any sport, is specific. There is no better way to get into shape for playing basketball than to play basketball or to practice the type of movements that basketball players use in a game. Basketball players need to use quick bursts of speed and side-to-side and up-and-back movements. In the preseason and during regular season drills, the coach should have his players practice moves in the manner mentioned above instead of merely running laps around a track or in a gym. Not only will it be more interesting for the players, but it will do a superior job of building endurance and strength in the players for playing basketball. The coach may have his players sprint for 20 to 30 yards and then do quick side to side movements; then sprint for another 20 to 30 yards and then perform quick up and back motions; sprint for another 20 to 30 yards and then reverse their direction quickly and repeat for several times. Utilizing this method of training will better condition players for the game of basketball than will the running of laps or running for long distances. It now appears that some form of interval training, adopted for the specific demands of the particular sport, is the best general method of conditioning.

The ability to do sustained work for a particular muscle group is another form of endurance. To build endurance in a particular muscle group, necessitates that many repetitions are done against a low resistance. The development of strength for his players in particular muscle groups is usually of great interest to the basketball coach.

For instance, many coaches like to attempt to improve their players' jumping ability, or their ability to grab rebounds with authority. This type of strength development should be done according to the specific task to be performed. In jumping, it is the plantor flexor group of the foot and the knee extensor group that needs to be developed. Strength is best developed by requiring fewer repetitions against a heavier resistance than is true with speed. The overload principle must also be followed to achieve maximum results. This means that the development of strength is dependent upon increasing the resistance that the muscles must overcome.

Despite the recent isometric fad, it is generally believed that participation in isotonic exercises is more beneficial to the development of strength over the long run. There are several reasons that may be offered in support of this concept. First, the use of isometrics appears to contribute very little toward the development of circulo-respiratory fitness, while the opposite is true with isotonic exercises. Second, the use of isometric exercises does not develop as much strength in the muscle as does isotonic. Third, isometric exercises are only beneficial for use in building strength at the limb angle at which they are practiced. For these reasons it is generally believed that an isotonic weight training program is superior to an isometric program. Many coaches, however, have had great success using a combination of the two exercise programs.

Coaches should realize that players who run long distances will develop circulo-respiratory endurance, but probably at the expense of the development of movements involving speed and quickness. This is especially true for tall or heavy players who need speed as much as they do endurance. To have these tall boys run cross country may retard their development of quick movement and ability to exert short bursts of speed. For other players, the harm is probably not so great as to be outweighed by the many benefits derived from participation in long distance running (but only in off- and preseason). Interval training may accomplish the required endurance goals as well as provide beneficial strength development exercise.

The preseason conditioning program should be quite different from the in-season conditioning program. Weight training and large doses of distance running should be done prior to the opening of the regular season. Most coaches prefer to have their players start in on a conditioning program when school opens in the fall and follow it until the regular season starts in December. They then often have them participate in the conditioning program again in the spring months before school is dismissed for the summer vacation. During the season many coaches prefer to use participation in drills on the basketball floor to maintain the conditioning that the players developed during the fall months. Many coaches have the players cease all weight lifting once the competitive season starts. It might be that some isometric work done in pairs may be beneficial to the players. It should be emphasized again that the drills used should contain the kinds of movement that take place in a basketball game. In only this way will they be of maximum benefit to the player.

There are many aids that the coach can use to develop strength and endurance in his players. Some of the more familiar ones in current use are weighted shoes, ankle weights, weighted vests, rebounding machines, jump ropes, and obstacle courses. Many of these devices should not be used during the playing season. Indiscriminate and purposeless use of them may result in little benefit accruing to the players.

A Pre-season Conditioning Basketball Program for College Players*

All players not competing in other fall sports will participate in the schedule of activities as contained below. The program will begin on a Monday, exactly four weeks before the commencement of the first official day of practice. It will end on the Friday before the opening of the initial day of

*An actual program used by a coach at a large university.

practice. The participants will take part in a total of twenty (20) sessions. Each session will be supervised by the student managers of the team. On the first day, the players will follow the workout and participate in the following exercises as outlined herein.

1. 5 gassers (32 seconds)
2. 5 bleacher leaps
3. 60 seconds of touching the backboard (use of 2 hands with standard ankle weights attached)
4. Big men–do 60 seconds of whirligig with standard weighted vest
5. Guards–do 60 seconds of ball handling
6. 1 hour scrimmage will be held.

1. Gassers

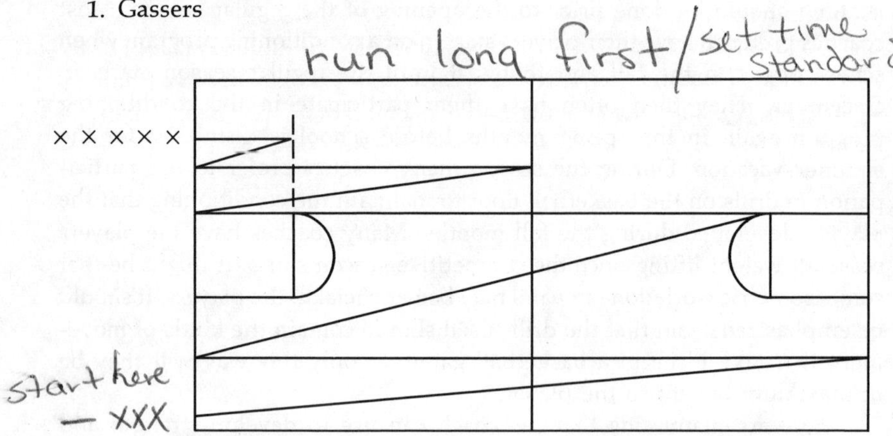

Begin at one endline, sprint to near foul line, thence back to original endline, on to center court line, then back to the original endline, then to other free throw line, back to other endline, return to far end, then back to original endline. Each complete circuit must be done in 32 seconds with a 30 second rest permitted between each complete run. The number of completed runs will be increased each day. Thus, on the 20th day, 25 will have been accomplished.

2. Bleachers

This must be adjusted to fit the facilities. The players run 5 laps around the entire gymnasium on the first day. These laps are increased one for each day for the duration of the 20 days.

3. Touching Backboard

Player stands directly under the background and jumps up as high as possible touching the board with both hands. He does this in as continuous a motion as possible without appearing to stop between jumps. He uses weights attached to his ankles. The drill lasts for 60 seconds.

4. Whirligig

Player stands directly under the basket with a ball in one hand. He hooks a shot one way, rebounds, then hooks the other way and rebounds. He does this in a continuous motion without stopping. He wears a weighted vest. The drill lasts for 60 seconds.

5. Ball Handling

Guards take part for 60 seconds in ball handling, participating in specific drills. Drills are those such as slapping the ball, executing a figure eight, going around the middle, rhythm of movement with the ball, etc.

6. Scrimmage

Players divide up into two teams and play for approximately 60 minutes. This time will be decreased as workouts become more intense. No supervision is permitted except that of the student managers.

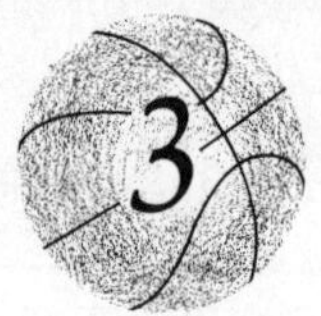

Formation of Team Offenses and Defenses

Individual Player Offense

The skills used by a player in making his individual offensive moves are many and varied. In this section an attempt is made to present selected offensive maneuvers, but not all of those known to and utilized by basketball players. Many other offensive skills and moves are discussed in the sections on dribbling, shooting, passing, and movement fundamentals.

A great deal of time is spent by most players perfecting offensive skills, especially during informal practice time. However, very little time is actually devoted to utilizing these skills in offensive maneuvers. Also, too little is understood by the players about the strategy involved in offensive maneuvering. The first items to be discussed here are the principles of individual offensive maneuvering.

PRINCIPLES CONNECTED WITH INDIVIDUAL OFFENSIVE MANEUVERING

1. Offensive maneuvers should be attempted to force the defensive player into a position of disadvantage.
2. Offensive maneuvers should not often be predetermined but rather they should be initiated in reaction to cues received from the defensive player (position, attitude, degree of concentration, etc.)
3. The offensive player in his maneuvers should attempt to capitalize on his offensive strengths.
4. The good offensive player normally should shoot or move quickly before the defensive man is prepared for his action.

5. Individual offensive maneuvers should be continuous and purposeful. The offensive player should not hesitate but should be daring in his maneuvers.

6. The good offensive player uses the dribble wisely and never aimlessly and carelessly.

7. When not in possession of the ball, the good offensive player must be continuously in motion in order to keep his defensive man occupied. This, among other things, prevents the defensive man from sagging off to guard other offensive players.

The purpose of any offensive maneuver is to attempt to force the defensive player into a *position of disadvantage.* This position of disadvantage of course is a relative term, because what might be a position of disadvantage in one situation might not be in another. For example, the offensive player might want to get the defender's body weight back toward his heels so that an outside shot might be attempted under the most favorable conditions possible. On the other hand, the offensive player might want to maneuver so that the defender raises his center of mass just enough so that an offensive drive toward the basket can be initiated without difficulty. Also, an offensive maneuver might cause a shift of body weight to be made by a defensive player in a given desired direction. This shift of body weight (backward or forward) might allow the offensive player enough time to drive toward the basket in the opposite direction from the weight shift. He might also take a quick dribble and get off a shot by moving in the opposite direction from the weight shift of the defensive players and toward the basket. It must be kept in mind that these examples involving change in the defensive player's positions could be shown to be of advantage to the defensive player(s) under certain circumstances. However, the important point to remember is that the offensive player must be able to recognize almost instantaneously that the defender is at a disadvantage, from his point of view and then he must attempt immediately to take advantage of the situation. It becomes obvious therefore that the attention of the offensive player must be directed toward the body position and body movements of the defender. In turn he must concentrate so that these momentary positions of defensive disadvantage are instantaneously recognized and responded to without hesitation.

Another thing to remember is that the offensive player usually should not move into the one-on-one situation with a preconceived detailed idea about what plans to use. That is, he should not have said to himself that under these circumstances I will drive to my right and attempt a jump shot. A predetermined idea about the move to use in any given situation may backfire because the defender may be able to move to an advantageous position to counter the preplanned movement. Instead of deciding beforehand what he will try, the offensive player should maneuver according to the continuous information that he receives by his recognition of the faults of the body positions and movements made by the defender. Hand and feet positions, his closeness in distance to the offensive player, and his weight shifts may all serve as cues for the offensive player to respond to advantageously. He reacts to these cues by maneuvering in such a manner as to take advantage of the information that he receives. For example, the offensive player might make a jab step toward the defender which forces the defender to move his front foot backward and shift his weight somewhat backward while dropping his hands down to his side. The offensive player can then bring his foot back more quickly than the defensive man can move his foot back to the starting position. The offensive player may now attempt a shot because the cues he has received tell him that the offensive player may well have a difficult time recovering in sufficient time to thwart his effort. If, when the shooting action has begun, the defender makes a last ditch successful effort to quickly shift his weight forward and upward in an attempt to stop the shot, the offensive player can receive this information and react to it. He may do this by changing the intended shooting movement and make an easy drive around the already over-committed defender. Years of practice and experience will enable the offensive player to react more quickly to such situations with less and less input information. He will learn to recognize that a slight movement in a given direction means that the defender may have committed himself ultimately to move in that direction. This slight cue allows him to react quickly without having to wait to see the entire movement unfold. This is one of the greatest advantages that experienced players have over the novice players.

The offensive player should attempt to capitalize on his particular offensive strengths. This is not to say that he should have predetermined the offensive maneuvers he will use, but rather that he should at every opportunity force the defensive player to respect his best moves. By way of illustration, if a player is a good jump shooter, he should usually make the defensive player defend against that shot before he tries other offensive possibilities. When in the mind of the player there is a doubt as to the possible success of certain moves, it is usually best to challenge the defender with his strongest moves. If an offensive player is able to move well to his right, he may find that a defender is overplaying him toward that direction. However, he usually should not immediately capitulate on this information by attempting to move to his left. Rather, he should patiently wait until he can utilize to the fullest extent this information. Too many young players get stopped at the outset of a game and never thereafter really make a concerted effort to utilize their strongest offensive moves, but often rely on those that are less effective for them.

While shooting skills are presented rather completely in another section, it is considered important to summarize the implication of their use in this section. The good offensive player must be able to shoot quickly but accurately at that moment when there is a defensive lapse created by his opponent, or when there is a momentary half-step of freedom developed by a good screen set by a teammate. He also should shoot with courage and with confidence. These two qualities would seem at first glance to be those found on two different sides of the same coin. However, if a player has confidence in his ability to shoot well, he should have the aggressive courage to take advantage of this ability. The good shooter reflects a picture of concentration. He shuts out all extraneous noises and movements that are not important to the immediate act. He focuses intently on his target. Concentration is one of the factors found most in the differences between the average and good shooter.

Individual offensive maneuvers should also be purposeful and continuous. They should be purposeful in the sense that every movement is made with the intention of contributing to the ultimate offensive act of shooting. Extraneous movements that do not directly contribute to the placing of the defender in a position of disadvantage should be eliminated. The movements should also be continuous yet fluid. The player should not make one feint and then stop before initiating the next one. He should execute one feint followed by another in a connected, purposeful pattern. It is often the use of a pattern of continuous feints that causes the defender to make a defensive mistake and thus the offensive player is permitted to score.

The good offensive player will use the dribble in a wise manner, that is, he will conserve his dribble until he can put it to good use. There is an old adage in basketball that states: "Don't put the ball down in a dribble unless you have some place to go." This simply means that the dribble should not be used unless the offensive player is ready to make a purposeful movement. The exception to this might be the offensive player who is attempting to move into a more effective offensive position from the controlled dribble. However, experience dictates that this type of player is the exception rather than the rule. Young players especially should be warned to conserve their dribble until they can put it to use as a real part of their offensive maneuver. A player should dribble the basketball on only five occasions: (1) When driving to the basket, (2) when attempting to get into a better position to pass the ball, (3) when getting out of trouble, (4) when bringing the ball down the floor, (5) when maintaining possession of the ball for a given time.

There is perhaps more of an opportunity for a player to be creative in developing individual offense moves than is possible in any other phase of the game. The number and types of maneuvers that might be used by players are virtually limitless. With this concept in mind, it might be of

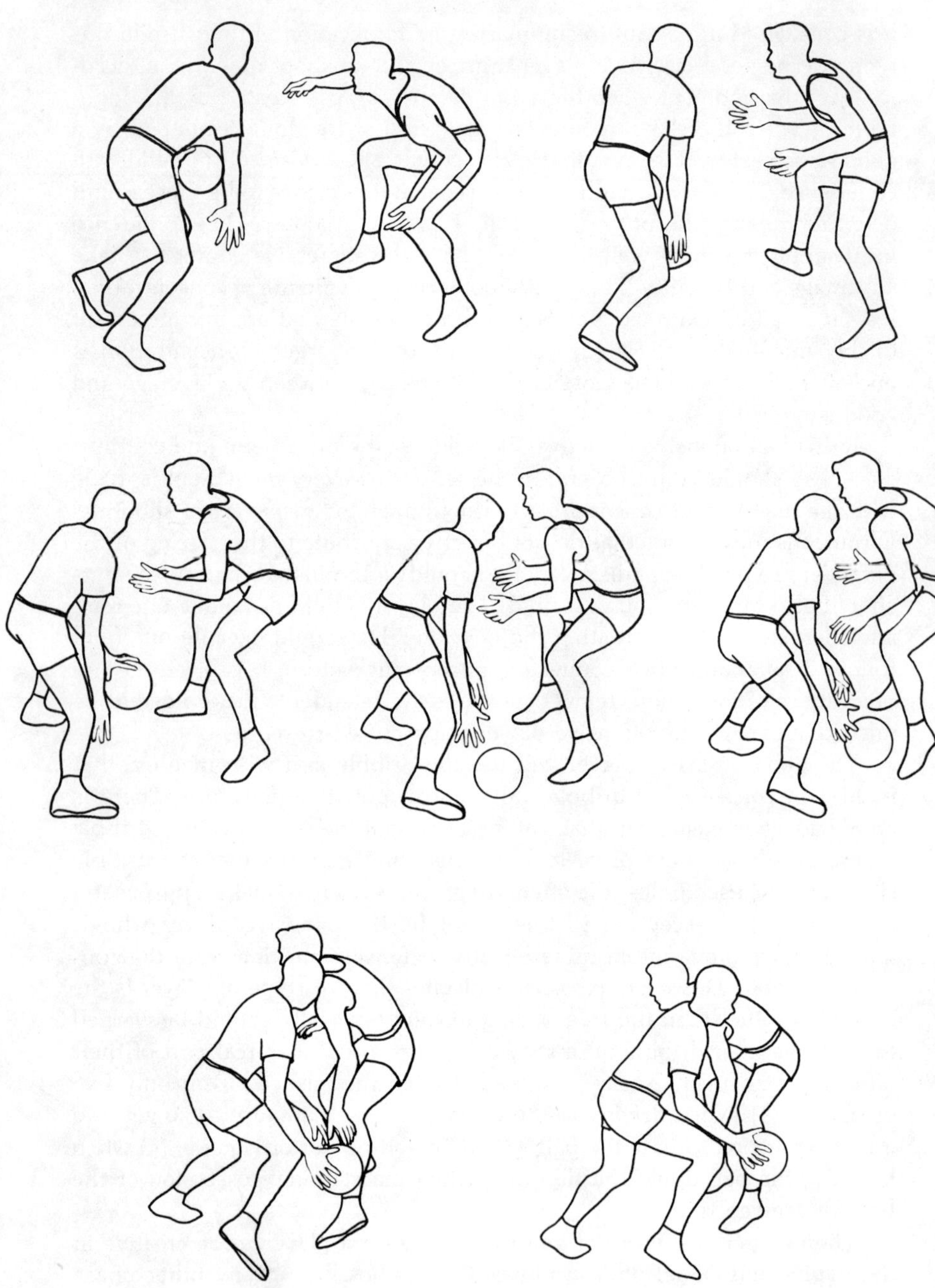

A change-of-hands dribble used against defensive player.

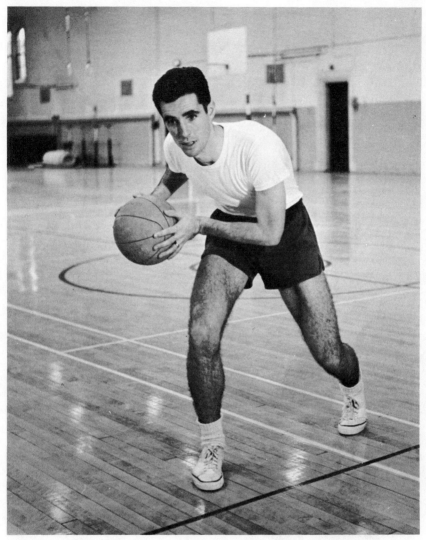

The jab step.

value to mention a few of the more commonly used offensive maneuvers. One successful maneuver used by players is to first place the ball high over their heads. If the defender does not come up quickly to counter this move, then the offensive player takes a shot from this position. If the defender does come up quickly to counter the move, he will normally have to raise his center of mass to do so. This will usually make him vulnerable to a

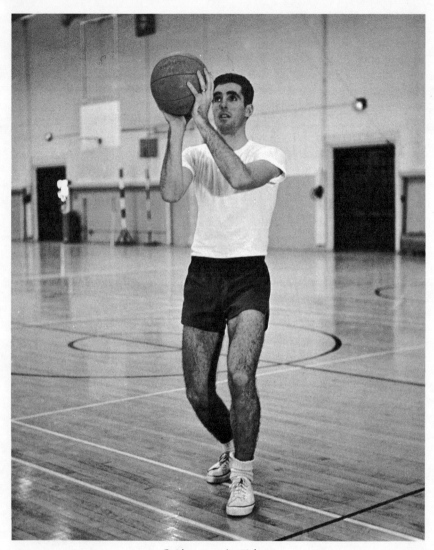

Quick recovery from jab step.

drive toward the basket being made by the offensive player. Another common maneuver is the use of the jab step. The jab step (short step) should be made directly at the defender's hip. If he does not immediately react to this movement by moving backward, then the offensive player may drive around him easily. If he reacts quickly to counter this movement, then a number of alternate possibilities are available. The offensive player might use a cross over step and drive by the defender in a new direction, or he might bring the lead foot back to its original position and take a quick outside shot. The rocker step is also often used and is a continuation of the jab step. It involves jabbing with a foot and bringing the foot back to its original position, then repeating it quickly to establish an offensive advantage. From the rocker step movement, a player can drive directly toward the basket, cross over and drive, rock back and shoot, or shoot from the jabbed step position. Another good offensive maneuver for the player to use is for him to fake a move with the ball instead of with the feet. An

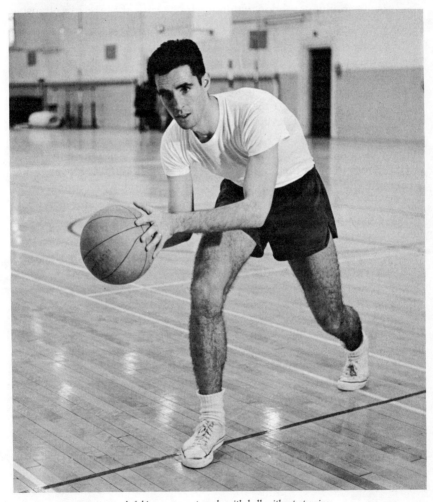

A faking movement made with ball without stepping.

effective fake to make is for the player to move the ball directly at but not against the face of the defender. This most often brings about a reflexive movement on the part of the defender. This reflexive action results in him ducking his head to get it out of the way of the ball. If the fake produces the reflexive action as described, then the offensive player may either shoot or drive toward the basket as he may choose because he has clearly established an offensive advantage.

Unfortunately, many players believe that individual offensive moves have to cease once they have passed the ball to a teammate. Nothing could be further from the truth. When not in possession of the ball, the good offensive player is in continuous motion within the framework of the team's offensive pattern. The most serious mistake that an offensive player makes is to stand still and watch his teammate maneuver. The offensive player can screen, he can cut for the basket, he can maneuver for position near the basket, or he can feint his opponent out of position in the anticipation of receiving a pass from a teammate. While doing all of these moves, the player continues to be an offensive threat. Fans are often amazed at the number of points scored by certain players even though they seemingly do not possess great offensive finesse. In the vast majority of cases, these players score because they are in continuous motion and always are on the move and on the watch in an attempt to be in the "right place at the right time." There is no other aspect of individual offense that needs as much constant prompting on the part of the coach as does the admonition that a successful scorer must be in continuous motion when he is without the ball.

Individual Player Defense

It is somewhat difficult to isolate principles of defense that belong only to a category known as individual defense. This is true because what is done in individual defense is necessarily conditioned by the defensive strategy employed by the team. Nevertheless in this section an attempt is made to mention those aspects of defense that are individual in nature as contrasted with those considered to be a part of team defense. However, variations in individual defense that are done primarily because they are team-oriented are also cited here. No attempt is made to examine the latter in detail. Also, individual defensive moves made primarily by a player performing in a man-to-man style of play are presented. Play in a zone defensive formation is similar but less exacting. This is because the individual player in such a style focuses attention primarily on the position of the ball and not on the man.

PRINCIPLES OF INDIVIDUAL DEFENSE

1. Playing good defense in a competitive situation is more a matter of attitude, desire, and concentration than it is proper execution of skills.
2. The main purpose of individual defense is to contain the man who has the ball and to prevent him and the offensive team from scoring.
3. Individual defense can be aided by the use of a mechanically sound stance.
4. Variations in the defensive stance used may depend upon the immediate situation and the planned team strategy.
5. The use of proper eye focus and concentration are essential to being a good defensive player.
6. The manner in which the first defensive stride is taken as the offensive player moves and the angle of pursuit used are fundamental to displaying good defensive play.
7. The footwork used by the defensive player should be continuously altered by the needs of the situation.

The movement skills used in individual defense are not particularly difficult to perform, yet to react immediately and effectively to maneuvers used by the offensive player may take years to master. Playing good defense in a competitive situation then seems to be more a matter of attitude, desire, and concentration than it is proper execution of skills. Learning defense, then, often becomes more a matter of motivation than of mechanics. Since this psychological aspect of defense is largely a team matter, it is considered in detail in the section on team defense. The discussion here will be limited to a presentation of the mechanics used in playing individual defense.

Since the purpose of individual defense is to contain the man with the ball, he and the offensive team must be prevented from scoring. This objective is largely accomplished on an individual basis by maintaining proper defensive position between the man with the ball and the basket, and by making it as difficult as possible for the offensive player to attempt to get off a good shot. The maintenance of a good defensive position is predicated upon the defensive man making proper movement responses to cues given to him by the maneuvers of the offensive player. Interpreting the cues correctly and responding properly are the cornerstones of good defensive play.

In order to move in the most effective manner the defensive player must first assume a proper defensive stance. It must be remembered that there are some aspects in connection with the defensive stance which are virtually universally adhered to in most situations regardless of the conditions. Thus, generally speaking, the stance initially selected is a compromise between stability and instability, (position for moving quickly in any given direction).

The stance must be a stable one so that a slight reaction (counteraction) by the defensive player to a false move by the offensive player will not throw the defensive player off balance. Increased stability (balance or equilibrium) is achieved by widening the base of support and lowering the center of gravity. Stability can be considered to be in direct proportion to the vertical and horizontal distance the center of gravity is from the base of support. The feet (often in a stride position) are usually spread a distance just beyond the width of the shoulders which should provide a wide enough base of support. The knees are flexed to an angle somewhere between 90 and 120 degrees. This should lower the center of gravity sufficiently to provide the necessary stability. If the defender increases the angle of knee flexion, thus lowering farther the center of gravity, he will gain additional stability but it will be at the expense of mobility. To insure that he may move quickly, the defender must compromise between stability and mobility. The amount of mobility indicated depends upon the needs of this situation and this in turn determines the width of the foot spread and the knee flexion used as mentioned above.

Another aspect of the stance that should be mentioned is the position of the trunk. The trunk should normally be held erect. This enables the defender to be able to move quickly in any given direction, forward, backward, or upward. The player who assumes a stance with a forward, backward, or sideward trunk lean will increase the ability to move in one specific direction, but will greatly decrease the ability to move in any other direction. However, since the defender does not often have the advantage of knowing in what direction the offensive man will move, he must be prepared to move in any given direction. This is the reason that the defensive player assumes a stance which makes him appear to be in a simulated sitting position.

Aside from adherence to the desired general mechanics of the defensive stance mentioned above, it is possible for a player to vary his stance in many ways to combat specific defensive situations. There seem to be three basic defensive stances used by most players, namely, the parallel stance, the stride stance, and the fencer's stance. The parallel stance, with the feet placed apart and directly across from each other, is best suited for use in lateral movement across the floor. In the stride stance, or boxer's stance as it is also termed, the feet are spread apart with one foot placed in front of the other. This stance is best suited for diagonal movement especially in the rear direction. This foot stance seems to be the most popular one with players and coaches, and is often considered to be the most comfortable and is a well-suited stance for use in countering offensive maneuvers. The fencer's stance is like the stride stance in that the feet are apart and one is forward and one is back. However, the fencer's stance differs from the stride stance in that the feet

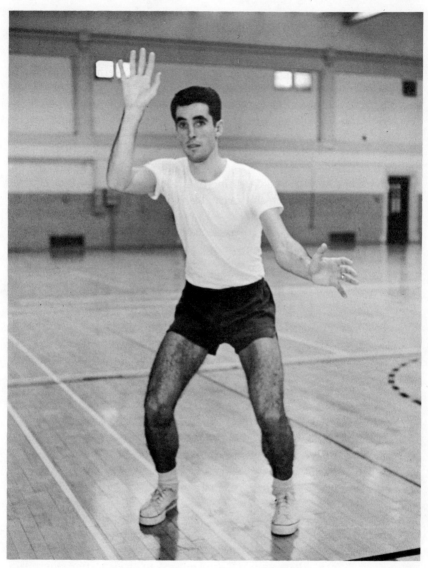

Parallel defensive stance—a simulated sitting position.

of the defensive player are not placed in the same direction. The back or rear foot is turned sideward to give a larger base from which force may be imparted. The front foot is pointed forward and is placed directly in front of the back foot. This latter feature also distinguishes this stance from the

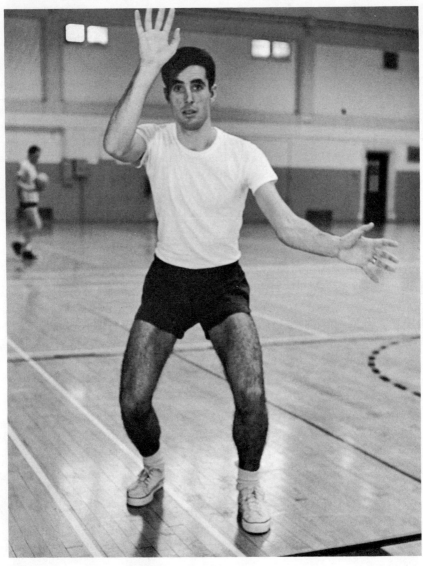

Boxer's stance.

others. The player who uses the fencer's stance is particularly suited for making quick forward and backward movements. But he has poor lateral stability and mobility.

The position of the hands must also be considered in discussing defensive stances. However, this is often an area where great disagreement exists as

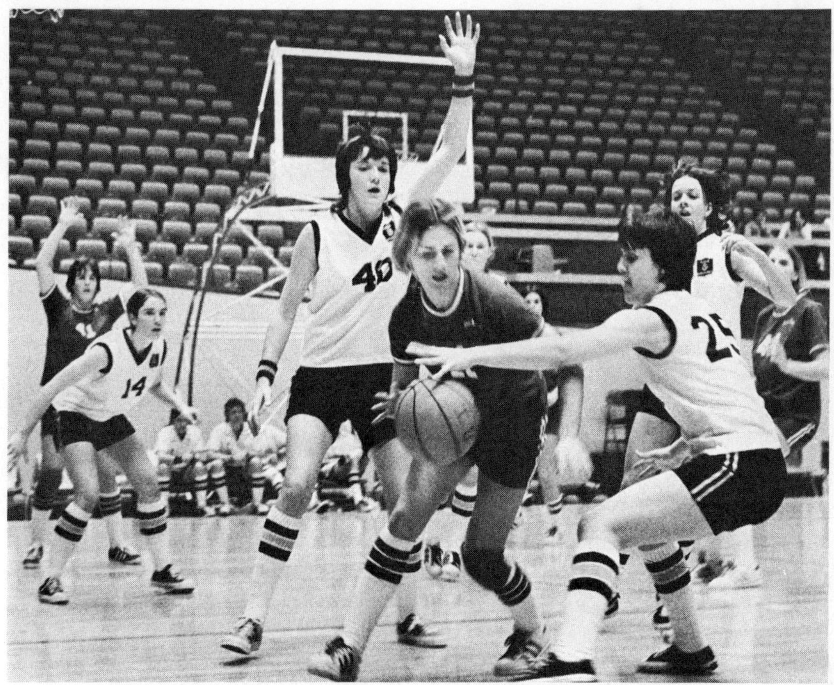

Trapping from the rear and in front. Note the stances of each defensive player (also see p. 160).

to the proper hand positions to use. It is agreed that the hands must be positioned to provide the most effective counter to the possible moves that might be made by the offensive player. For example, if the offensive player is holding the ball above his head, then the hands of the defensive player must be held high. Likewise, if the ball is held low, the hands must counter this threat by being placed in a low position. Against a non-driving jump shooter both hands should be raised to an overhead position. Most offensive players begin their moves with the ball placed near their belt. (This ball position is the basic position used when the offensive player prepares to dribble.)

The defensive player, to defend properly in this situation, should keep the hand nearest the shooting hand high so as to hinder a possible shot being made at the basket. The other hand opposite from the opponent's shooting hand should be kept in a low position to protect against the possible change of direction being made by the offensive player by his foot movements and/or by dribbling. Regardless of the initial hand positions used by the defensive player, he must learn to move his hands and arms through their full range of motion without appreciably shifting his center of mass.

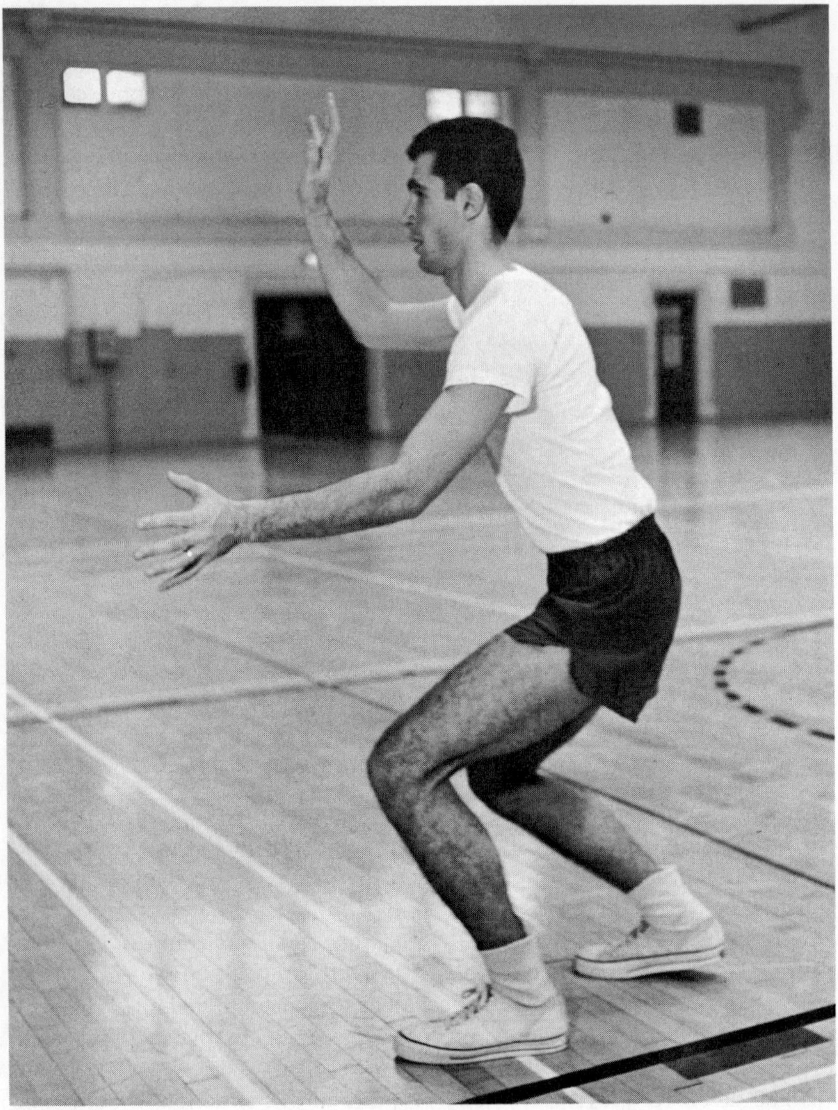

Defensive stride stance—one hand up, the other low.

Thus he keeps as much stability as possible and still offers as much interference as he can.

The proper body weight distribution to be used over the feet is another often controversial issue. Like hand positioning, body weight distribution is determined by the needs of the situation. It is probably influenced most by how close the defensive player is to the offensive player. Provided he is about 3 feet from the offensive player, most coaches would want their defensive player to distribute his weight evenly on his feet. Some coaches prefer to have their defensive player start off by being very close to the offensive player in order to harass him and attempt to force him into making an error. In this situation the body weight of the defensive player is placed more on the heels than the toes. It is strongly recommended that the defender in most situations be close enough to the offensive man who has the ball so that he can bother him with the use of his hands without having to shift his weight forward. The vast majority of defensive mistakes occur as the defender shifts his weight forward to harass the offensive player. He then cannot recover his position nor react quickly enough to foil an offensive player's moves made toward the basket.

Stance may also be considered in terms of the position of total body rather than just the position of the feet. This is involved with team and even individual defensive strategy and may seem to be more properly considered in the section on team defense. However, a description of some of the possibilities in this connection will suffice for purposes of this discussion on individual defense. Players can, by positioning their body in a certain way, discourage movement in a given direction. Most high school players, for example, should often overplay almost a half-man toward the shooting hand of their opponent. They would thus force him to use his non-preferred hand or to move in a direction where the use of the preferred hand would be less effective. Some coaches prefer to force all offensive movement toward the middle of the floor. Regardless, movement of the offensive player in the desired direction is accomplished by the placing of the body in a position to make it easy for the offensive player to move in that direction.

Proper eye focus and concentration are closely related in that proper eye focus seems to be a prerequisite for developing effective concentration. The defensive player guarding the player with the ball should focus his eyes on the center of mass of the opponent, which is most often near the belt buckle. When a true movement is initiated by the offensive player the center of gravity must move. A false cue, such as an arm movement or head fake, does not appreciably effect the center of mass. The expert defender eventually learns to disregard these false cues somewhat, and to react only to a true movement that involves a change in the position of the center of mass. The defensive player may have to move his hands to counter the hand positions of the offensive player, but this does not need to involve much movement of his center of mass. While focusing the eyes on the center of mass of the offensive player, the peripheral field of vision should not be neglected entirely. The defensive player should also be aware of movement made in the immediate area especially any made by potential screeners. It must be emphasized that the defensive player's primary responsibility is to contain the man with the ball. He should never shift his eye focus in detecting a potential screen to the extent that he fails to react quickly to a true offensive movement made by the man he is assigned to guard.

Defensive players who are not directly involved with guarding the man with the ball should focus their attention on something that is not in their immediate area of the floor. By focusing on something somewhat farther away, they increase the range of their peripheral vision and they can be more aware of the total movement made by the players on the floor. If they focus their attention on a player or a spot on the floor that is some distance from them, they will probably make maximum use of their viewing possibilities.

With the use of proper eye focus the player can concentrate effectively on his defensive task. Great defensive players are those who concentrate intensely which enables them to be able to react quickly to the visual cues that they receive from the maneuvers of the offensive player. Concentration is not a phenomenon nor is it innate. It is a skill attained by devoting much time and effort to its achievement.

Upon the initiation of movement by an offensive player, the defensive player's objective becomes that of cutting-off this movement and stopping it as far away from the basket as is possible. For this reason, the first step that the defensive player takes becomes extremely important. It must be taken quickly; it must be a long step; it must be a low step; and it must be taken in the right direction. Once he decides where his opponent is going, the defensive player must move as quickly as possible. A powerful pushoff made with the foot away from the direction of the offensive movement should be accompanied by a vigorous reaching out with the other foot and leg toward the anticipated direction of the offensive movement. As previously stated, this step must be quite long and kept as close to the floor as possible. Also, the step should be taken in a direction that will cause the defensive player to cut off his opponent rather than follow him. The faster the offensive player is or the more of a jump he gets on the defensive player, the larger the angle must be for the defensive player to reach an acceptable cut-off spot. If the proper angle is not chosen, then the defensive man will not have enough time to move across the path of the offensive man. Thus he may end up being on the side of the offensive man rather than in front of him as he drives toward the basket. It should be obvious from this discussion that the success or failure of the defensive cut-off procedures depends on the effectiveness of the first steps taken by the defender.

Normally, these first few steps should be gliding ones that do not involve crossing the feet and legs over one another. The center of mass should not be raised substantially during the first step, due to the great length of the step. However, when the feet come together to begin the second step the center of mass will be raised somewhat. In succeeding steps it should remain somewhat above the level it was during the beginning guarding position and during the first stride. There are instances when a particularly good offensive movement may have left the defender so called "flatfooted." When this occurs, the defender must react quickly to recover his defensive position by selecting a larger angle at which to execute the move to cut off the offensive player. In this situation he may have to use a cross-over starting step and continue such steps in running to the desired spot. Gliding steps are not executed as fast as true running steps. Thus the defender may forsake the use of gliding steps to achieve his purpose in this instance.

The defensive player must not fail to remember that his hands still have a defensive function to perform once an offensive movement has been initiated. The trailing hand should be carried low to guard against the possibility of a change of direction dribble or low pass being used. The lead arm can be used to protect against a potential shot or pass being attempted. It can be also used to harass the dribble moves. A common error made on defense is to attempt to harass the dribbler with the trailing hand rather than with the leading hand. This error in turn creates two problems. First, it may often cause unnecessary fouling to take place because the trailing shoulder may bump the offensive player. This shoulder has been rotated inwardly so that the trailing arm can reach across to harass the dribbling action. It often comes in contact with the trailing leg or hip of the dribbler. Second, this move makes the defensive player vulnerable to a reverse dribble action. This results because the entire upper part of the defender's body has been turned sideward to permit him to reach toward the offensive player with the trailing hand.

Defense then may be stated as largely a matter of concentration and desire. The defender should be "offensively" minded in that he must take the play away from the offensive player rather than waiting and only reacting to his offensive maneuvers. Also, the defensive player should present a challenge to his opponent by constantly changing his tactics. The pressure must be continuous without relaxation in order not to give the offensive player an opportunity to reverse the situation and put the defender on the "defensive." In order to achieve this goal the defender must make false moves and feints much in the same manner as that done by the offensive player.

Selecting the Players on the Squad

The selection of the members of a basketball squad is one of the most important tasks that a coach must perform. However, some aspects of it may be very crucial, difficult and even unpleasant. For example, it can be unpleasant if the coach has been placed in the position of having to cut or drop a boy from the squad whom he knows wants very badly to be a member of the team. The coach may like him very much, but he believes he just does not meet the necessary standards decided upon as criteria for team membership. Final selection of the squad members is a crucial task because it limits the number of players that the coach has available. It somewhat determines the physical and psychological makeup of his team. Furthermore, selection can prove to be a difficult duty, especially when a coach must decide between several boys of seemingly equal ability to fill the last remaining positions on the squad. It is not usually difficult to select the first 8 or 10 players who will be on the team, but to determine the last 4 to 6 to be on the squad is often a nearly impossible task. The selection of the members of the team, then, is always crucial, most always difficult, and not always pleasant, yet it must be done. The information in this section contains suggested guiding principles that might be used to help the coach make the wisest decisions possible in this matter.

SUGGESTED PRINCIPLES FOR USE IN SELECTING TEAM MEMBERS

1. Coaches should first define the qualities that they feel are essential and desirable to have in squad members.
2. Coaches should then determine the criteria by which the prospective team members will be selected.
3. Basketball skills tests are considered to be of limited value as a means of aiding the coach in the selection of team members.
4. Prospective team members should be observed in competitive situations.
5. Every available bit of information about each prospective player should be collected to add to the validity of the selection process.
6. There is no substitute for the worth of the evaluation of an experienced observer.
7. The opinions of several experienced observers is probably the most valid measure of judging playing ability.
8. The final decision on determining squad membership should be made by the coach(es) only.

The first step to take in the selection process is for the coach to determine those qualities that he feels are essential for becoming squad members. These may be physical qualities such as height, skills, unique abilities such as great proficiency in shooting, and/or attitude qualities such as the willingness to discipline oneself to a high degree. (This may involve selection of a certain kind of player for each position.) The coach must then determine those few qualities that he feels are absolutely essential for becoming a team member. Next he must list those qualities that he feels are desirable, but not necessarily essential. These procedures, if followed, will result in a rank order of certain qualities being made by the coach. These could be used as the yardsticks by which the prospective team members will be judged and selected to be members of the team.

The coach must next decide on how large in number he wants his squad to be. He may let the quality of the prospective players determine to a degree that decision. Some coaches prefer to limit squad membership to a total of 12 because they find it easier to work with this number of players. A few coaches select the best 8 to 10 players for their playing squad and then 4 to 5 more players are selected as "holler" players. These latter are not necessarily the best players available, but ones who will be loyal to the team and will help preserve harmony. On the other hand, some coaches are much more flexible about this matter. They may keep up to 20 members on their squad during those years when their player talent is of high quality. Regardless, this basic question about squad size should be answered before the selection process is begun.

The scores made on objective basketball skills tests are sometimes used to aid a coach in the selection of the members of a squad. At the present time this is not considered a good procedure; tests are not precise enough to be used for this purpose. The influence of the dispersion of any particular group upon the validity of the items used in any known test to measure a given group's ability in basketball is too great. The results from the administration of a skills test might be more profitably utilized to make a preliminary cut of a junior high group of prospective basketball players from 150 down to 50, but to cut a college squad from 30 down to 15 using the same skills test items or ones similar to them would be virtually useless. This is because the dispersion of ability is so much less with the college group than with the junior high group. Someday, some diligent and competent investigator might develop a test battery that could accurately predict basketball playing ability within a somewhat homogenous group, but no test exists today that even approaches this standard of predictive validity. This suggests that coaches should use this tool in a most limited way if they use it at all as a predictive procedure. Expert empirical judgment is the most valid procedure to use as of now.

All candidates for a team should be given a chance to perform in a competitive, full-court game situation. Some players perform well in half-court situations, while some are great practice shooters. Still others look very inept until they are involved in a full-court situation. The point to be made is that basketball is a game played in a full-court situation, and that there is no substitute for evaluating a boy under such conditions. A surprising number of players will actually perform quite differently in a full-court situation than they will in the half-court or one-on-one situations. Some will even be better and some will be worse in the full-court situation, but almost all will perform differently. The coach must be aware of the possibility of such variances occurring as he makes his evaluation of their playing ability. All available information known about the players should be used in the evaluative process. The more the coach knows about the players, the more valid his final choices will be. Such information can be of almost any kind in addition to their basketball playing ability; *i.e.* academic, social, home background, special interests, work capacity, tenacity, performance in other sports, performance in group situations, etc. Each bit of information known to the coach adds to the total picture he has of each individual. It will aid him in choosing those boys who best meet the criteria he has set as being essential and desirable.

The evaluation made by an experienced observer is invaluable. A corollary to this concept is that the opinions of two or three experienced observers are better than one. Probably the most reliable sources of information for the coach to make use of when final evaluation day arrives is the opinion of experienced observers. The coach should not be afraid to rely upon two or three close friends (basketball-wise individuals) whose judgment he respects and whose experiences might qualify them for this capacity when he selects his squad members. This is especially a good policy for a young coach to follow.

When all the information is collected and is digested, it remains for the coach to be the final sole agent in the decision making process. Perhaps, the task still remains just as difficult, just as crucial, and just as unpleasant as when this presentation began. Yet it is hoped that the coach will make use of some of the suggestions presented here so that the decisions he finally makes on who will be members of his basketball squad has supporting evidence.

Selecting the Starters

The more familiar a coach is with his players and their abilities, the more likely he is to induce a maximum performance from them on any given night. Therefore, it is important that the coach knows the physical capabilities of each player, that is, for example, the best jumper, the best dribbler, and the best free throw shooter. Likewise, as mentioned before, he should also know as much as he can about the personalities of the players; their academic interests; their home background; their social life; their vocational plans; and their religious beliefs. Most coaches are usually fully cognizant of these factors and the important role that they can play in their success as coaches. Furthermore, experience has revealed that there are often "competitive types" among the players and that in basketball, knowledge of the existence of these types on a team can be of great value. This knowledge can be of value in terms of planning for the entire season, and it can be of value in developing strategy for a given situation in any game on the schedule. Below are listed some of the more common "basketball types."

THE HOME FLOOR PLAYER

The home floor player is one who plays well before the friendly home crowd but does not perform well away from home. This type is more often found among the front line substitutes. The reason for this occurrence may lie in the fact that he is insecure, is in unfamiliar surroundings and/or needs friendly support to perform well.

THE THREE O'CLOCK SHOOTER

This type of player scores well in every practice, but is only a mediocre shooter in a game. The solution to the problem for this player can only be found by recreating as much as is possible the game atmosphere during practice sessions.

THE FRIDAY OR SATURDAY NIGHT PLAYER

This type of player is one who looks forward to playing in the games, but does not like to work in practice sessions. This type of player can have a very negative effect upon the attitude of a team.

THE ONE-ON-ONE OR TWO-ON-TWO PLAYER

This type of player will perform well during the one-on-one drills held early in the season and may also perform well during the two-on-two sessions. However, once the five-on-five practice drills begin his offensive potential is greatly reduced. The problem may lie in the fact that this type of player needs more room to maneuver, or that he just does not see more than 2 or 3 players at a time. He should be encouraged to limit the area in which he moves so as to more nearly create the game situation during practice. His problem may also stem from his inability to fit successfully into an offensive pattern, or to anticipate correctly the movements of his teammates.

THE SUCCESSFUL-FOR-A-FEW-MINUTES PLAYER

This type of player plays well for a few minutes, but his performance dwindles off rapidly when he gets a little tired. The problem may be just a case of poor conditioning, but it may stem from deeper physiological reasons. If a stepped up conditioning program does not correct the problem, then further medical assistance should be sought.

DEFENSIVE TYPES

Some players play lateral defense well but cannot play up and back defense effectively. Some players may blossom out into fine players with the introduction of a change in defensive formation, such as a change from a standard man-to-man defense to a pressing defense. Some players will play much better defense when challenged with a difficult individual assignment. Some players feel constrained when playing a tight zone defense and their performance may suffer. Some players may perform well as defensive guards, but are only mediocre as defensive forwards. The coach needs to know their abilities well enough to use them properly.

OFFENSIVE TYPES

A change in offensive procedures may bring out undiscovered abilities in certain players. Some players have great trouble limiting their movements so that they can play effectively in a precise, continuity offense. However, they may be fine passers and shooters when playing in a less confining offensive pattern of play. Some players perform best offensively when left entirely alone without any help being given them by their teammates. To set a screen for this type of player only hinders his potential. Other players may be extremely mediocre as one-on-one performers, but may turn out to be great shooters when given aid through the setting of screens.

Coaches should be constantly aware of such players and their possibilities as mentioned above. Their abilities and peculiarities may be seen in a practice session or in a game situation. Regardless, sooner or later many of these types will appear on the scene. How effectively they are utilized may be a determining factor in how successful the coach becomes.

Team Offenses

One of the important responsibilities of a basketball coach is to plan, select, mold, and solidify an offensive style of play to be used by the members of his team. At the outset it must be stated that in deciding on the offense he will use during a given season, the coach is influenced by many factors. Some of these influential factors are the quantity and quality of his players, the caliber of his opponents, the type of facilities available, and finally the extent of his background and experience. While some of these factors may be different for each individual, it is necessary that most of them be given consideration in the decision-making process concerning the team offensive pattern used during a given season.

PRINCIPLES OF TEAM OFFENSE SELECTION

1. It is usually a sound procedure for the coach initially to select for use by his players an offensive system with which he has had some experience as a player and coach.
2. The size of the home court and other courts in the conference may influence the offensive style of play decided upon for use by his players.
3. The offense should be selected to fit the specific players on the team and should permit them to take advantage of their strengths.
4. The offense should be planned with the experience and maturity of the present players kept in mind.
5. Consideration of the team defenses most likely to be met during the season should be recognized in the planning.
6. The philosophy of the coach in reference to his concepts of team and individual styles of play will influence the selection.
7. The tradition of the school and the particular experiences of the local fans should be considered, but should never dominate the final decision.

The coach should have confidence in the offensive pattern he selects and also confidence in his ability to teach it to his players. The younger coach usually selects an offense that he has had experience with in some capacity. He might modify an offensive style of play he has previously used, or one that he used as a player, but it would normally not be a good policy under this condition to attempt to develop an offensive style that is completely new to him. Once a coach has gained experience he may then want to experiment with other patterns of play, but a beginning coach may find it difficult to teach a new offense to his players. The primary reason for this statement is that the players will have only as much confidence in using the offense as the coach shows in teaching it to them.

The size and kind of courts encountered during a season are not usually big factors to consider, but they are still large enough ones to warrant consideration in planning a team's offensive style of play. A small home court may give the home team a decided advantage if they plan their offense to take advantage of it. However, it may become a disadvantage when the team travels away from home to play on larger courts. Small courts lend themselves well to the use of zone and pressing defenses, and offensive planning by a coach must take this into consideration.

The offense should fit the talents and abilities of a specific group of players. An attempt should not be made to fit the players to the offensive style selected. Teams composed of short (in stature) players may have to use fluid, continuity offenses, involving screening and cuts. Good player speed may also warrant the use of the fast break, while lack of speed may cause the coach to favor the use of a more controlled offense. Also, spot shooters should be taken advantage of by providing situations for them. Likewise, normally, the very tall player should be playing a style which allows him to be stationed near the basket. It is understood that the assessment of individual abilities is made in relation to the opponents' abilities. Members of a team may be quick in relation to other teams in a league, yet slow in comparison to top players. A team may have no player on it who is over 6 feet 5 inches in height yet the team height may be tall in comparison with the opponents' height.

The team offensive moves should be planned and selected with the experience and maturity of the players kept in mind. The more experienced the players, the more can be expected in the way of versatility of attack. They can learn more intricate team movements, and be expected to use more advanced individual moves. More allowance might be made for permitting individual deviations within the basic pattern. The younger, the less experienced the members of the team are, the stricter the adherence to a pattern, and use may be made of more formal screening situations. The younger, less experienced players, however, should not be expected to learn offensive team movements in one season which require split second timing and are composed of intricate movements.

The defenses that a coach expects to meet during a season should have influence on his offensive planning. If the majority of the opponents use zone defenses, then his planning must come up with an offense that is effective against zone defenses. If the teams his team plays against use aggressive man-to-man defenses, then cutting and screening offenses should be considered for use by his team. It is at this point that the speed and height of one coach's players in relation to that of the others becomes important in the ultimate selection of an offense.

The philosophy of the coach in reference to team and individual play may also influence the selection of the offensive pattern and the implementations he may introduce. The single post offense, for example, depends on fine teamwork most of the time for success. It involves the use of many screens and double cuts, and is one of the great team offenses now in use today. The single pivot offense may also be used to take advantage of the abilities of the tall, high-scoring center. The final selection then will depend to a great extent on the coaches personal basketball philosophy and also on his personnel. The same is true in regards to the fast break. The question of whether to use a fast break or not usually, in the final analysis, is decided by the coach's basic conceptions about how the game of basketball should be played and what player talents he has available.

It is probably as incorrect to ignore completely the basketball tradition of a school and the expressed views of the fans as it is to let them dominate the decision-making process on the selection of the offense. If a new coach installs a controlled offense in a school that has traditionally used a fast break, free lancing offense, he may end up with a dissatisfied audience as well as discontented players. These things should be considered, and if a change is deemed desirable, the public and players should be prepared for it and if possible, it should be brought about slowly rather than abruptly in most instances. Of course, nothing succeeds like success, and a few important victories along the way are the best way to change seemingly entrenched traditions. It is important, however, that the prospective basketball coach come to grips with some of the hard realities of his profession, and that if the players and crowd tend to be dissatisfied with the offensive system he selected, he may not remain as basketball coach very long in such a community.

The above factors should all be considered when the coach sits down to map out his offensive campaign for the coming season. Consideration of these factors will provide a good basis upon which he may build a framework of ideas. His final plans must be consummated with confidence and with a reasonable certainty that the decision is the right one. There are general characteristics of good offenses that may be identified and certain important principles of teaching an offense that must now be considered.

PRINCIPLES OF TEAM OFFENSE

1. Any system of play may be effective if the players and coach know it well and have confidence in using it.
2. The good offense can be modified so that it can be readily adapted for use against any type of defense.
3. The good offensive style is such that if the defense prevents one man from operating effectively, the entire offense is not rendered ineffective.
4. Good offensive team play helps maintain court balance so that the defense will not have a rebound or fast break advantage.
5. The use of a good offense provides a degree of latitude that permits free lancing within the framework of the basic pattern.
6. The good offensive pattern is not so intricate that the players have

great difficulty understanding and executing it, but has enough variations that it is adaptable yet not too easy to scout and defend against.

7. A balanced attack of shooting (long and short shots) as well as good defensive play is present in a good offense.

8. Good offensive play demands that all men are kept moving, especially those who are not directly involved with handling the ball.

9. The use of a good offense makes the defensive players stay where they belong and does not permit them to double team, or make counter-movements so that double team situations are involved.

10. The good offensive pattern does not call for the use of many difficult or unusual passes to be executed to make it effective.

With the use of any offensive style of play a team has a reasonable chance of being successful if the coach and players know it well and have confidence in using it. A team may offensively violate many of the principles presented here, and still have success because they believe in the offense they are using. This should not, however, be taken as a blanket approval of all offenses, and the suggestions offered here will, if used, other things being equal, tend to improve an existing offense or reveal characteristics of a good offense that might be considered in developing one.

The good offense provides variations that cause it to be adaptable for use against many defensive situations. The good offense can be used against a man-to-man and zone defenses with the use of only slight modifications. It has become increasingly more popular for a team to play a defensive style which permits them to switch from man-to-man to zone many times during a game. The good modern offensive team then cannot afford the luxury of using a separate offense against zone and man-to-man defenses. Instead it should have a style of offensive play that is readily adaptable for use against a zone defense and man-to-man defense as well.

The offense used by a good team does not depend upon the abilities of one man for its success. Therefore, a team using it is not completely thwarted when the defense successfully prevents one of its men from operating effectively. This is true especially in connection with the pivot man. Stopping the pivot man should not completely thwart the rest of the team's offensive play. It also may be true in relation to one of the guards on the team. While it is a good policy to have one guard who "quarterbacks" the offense, his role should not be such that a defense can thwart the entire team offense just by successfully containing him. The same principle holds true as it relates to the passing lanes. The success or failure of the offense used by a team should not depend upon the successful execution of a pass into a certain lane. For instance, many team offenses are initiated by a pass being made from a guard to a forward on the same side of the floor, but this should not be the only way in which the team might begin its offensive play. If the defensive player shuts off one important passing lane, then the team should have another secondary lane ready for use that is a part of the planned offense.

The team having a good offensive style of play maintains court balance. This prevents the defensive team from operating so that the players can rebound more effectively on one side of the backboard. Also it prevents them from easily initiating and completing fast breaks. Court balance should be maintained by the team at the initiation and completion of the offensive pattern. That is, a series of cuts and picks should not result in an extremely unbalanced offensive position on the court being made by the players. This principle also holds true because it is of great advantage to the offensive team to keep the defensive team spread out on the floor, thus keeping the passing and cutting lanes free for possible offensive thrusts being made by the players.

The completely free lance type of offense and the completely pattern type of offense are seldom used by teams in today's game of basketball. Instead, most coaches tend to prefer to use a basic pattern type of offense that has enough latitude in it so that individual players are permitted to improvise movements on their own within the basic pattern of play. This not only allows individual players to best utilize their individual abilities, but also presents the defensive team with a more difficult task; that is, they cannot always predict the movements that the players of the offensive team will make under given situations. It is also thought that the use of this type of offense is the most enjoyable one for the players to use, and, therefore, is best for maintaining a high level of player interest, morale, and enthusiasm. The successful use of a completely free lance type of offense requires that all of the players not only possess great individual skill, but are also adept at using great teamwork. On the other hand, the team using the completely pattern type of offensive style of play often fails to take advantage of defensive lapses. It can also be more easily stopped by defensive players who have scouted the moves of the players using this style and are able to anticipate their actions. Most coaches, therefore, prefer to have their team use an offense that utilizes the advantages and minimizes the disadvantages of each.

The good offensive pattern should not be so intricate that the players have great difficulty understanding and executing the moves in it. Yet, there should be enough variations that are adaptable to use against many defenses to justify its use. It should not be too easy to scout nor easy to defend against. The degree of intricacy that the offense possesses should be geared to the playing experience of the team members. An intricate offense which involves a series of screens and cuts should be attempted only by teams whose members have considerable experience, and who also have ample time to master the offense. It has been estimated that a minimum of two years is needed to master moves in such an offense. On the other hand, the offense should have enough variations that it is adaptable for use against many different types of defenses. For example, some teams that use many screens in their offensive play usually can be easily stopped by the use of a switching man-to-man defense. This of course should not occur. Their team offense should be such that certain variations are incorporated so that advantage can be taken of a team using a switching man-to-man defense.

The team using a good offensive pattern gets a balanced attack from its players of shooting over the defense as well as driving in for short shots. If this balance does not exist, then the defensive player can sag back and stop the driving, or he can play aggressively and stop the outside shooting attack. An adequate blend of outside shooting and driving toward the basket will help prevent the defense from setting itself to stop one style of scoring threat. Many players today have become convinced that they cannot often drive in close to the basket for the attempt at the short shot because of the presence of the tall defensive center. Therefore their team uses an offensive style that is designed solely to have them attempt the medium range jump shot. The players on a defensive team who have this information from scouting reports or from viewing the team's previous games can have their defensive guards play much more aggressively on the outside shooters than they would ordinarily if they felt that the drive for the short shot was a only frequent part of their offensive attack.

All players must keep moving, especially those who, if their offensive attack is to be effective, are not directly involved with handling the ball. The mark of a good basketball player is his ability to maneuver and keep in motion when he does not have the ball. The mark of a good offensive team is its ability to keep all five men in motion so that they are constant offensive threats, and thus engage the attention of defensive players at all times. If some players are permitted to just stand still when not directly involved with handling the ball, the defense will sag off the defensive players assigned to them and help out teammates who are directly engaged in guarding the offensive players with the ball. This is an aspect of offensive team play that is too often overlooked by many coaches.

The good offensive team must make the defensive team "play honestly." That is, the coach should check his offensive style to determine if there are any crucial spots in which the defensive team might use double-team tactics. If there are, the coach should make the necessary offensive adjustments to insure that the double-team maneuvers can be discouraged. Many defensive teams are successful because they allow certain players to "cheat" on their man and to help out elsewhere on the court against a stronger part of the offense. Thus, the coach should attempt to use an offense that discourages this type of "cheating" by maneuvering his players so that each defensive player feels that he must play his man "honestly" or risk giving up an attempted shot at the basket.

The effective use of an offense pattern should not mean that many difficult or unusual passes must be executed. While a lob pass or a difficult bounce pass may be utilized occasionally within the pattern of an offense, it is generally incorrect to have to rely on many such difficult passes for the efficient use of a pattern of play. The two-hand chest pass remains as the quickest and most accurate pass to use in most offensive situations. This pass should be used on every feasible occasion. Other passes should be used only when the two-hand chest pass cannot be delivered effectively. Occasionally the bounce pass made to a "backdoor" cutter or a lob pass made to a weakside cutter should be used, and as such should be considered as a main part of the offensive pattern. But, these passes are often difficult to execute and the defensive players always have a chance to intercept them. An offensive pattern to be effective should not depend on these passes as the basic ones or else its use will be hampered.

An attempt will now be made to present the main features and specific characteristics of several offenses. No attempt is made here to describe in detail all of the offensive patterns that are in current use. Rather it is hoped that the information presented of a sample of some basic "types" will serve as the foundation for the coach to use to develop his own particular style of offense that best suits his own needs. A rather detailed description of a number of selected offenses with accompanying diagramatic explanations appears in the appendix.

SINGLE POST OFFENSES

Teams using single post offenses have operationally two guards, two forwards, and a post man. (See discussion on post play, p. 114.) The distinguishing feature of this type of offense over others lies in how the post man is used. The coach who has a tall post man, who is a good scorer, may want to station him at a low post position. When a single post offense operates with a low post player, then the other players used in this offense are generally asked to pass the ball to this pivot man so that he may attempt as many shots as possible close to the basket. The low post player position is generally the poorest one to play in terms of the player being able to pass the ball off to teammates as they use cutting maneuvers while going by him. Teams using offenses of this type often have to use cuts between the guards and the forwards instead of those that go by the player.

Most typical of the single post offenses used by teams today is that one in which a medium high (lanewise) man stations himself to one side of the lane about halfway between the free throw line and the basket. From this position the man can be an offensive threat himself since he is within his shooting range. He may also act as a feeder to his teammates and as a post player in case double cuts are made by teammates as they go by him. While the low post man almost always plays and shoots with his back to the basket, the medium high post man can turn and face the basket when he receives the ball so he may shoot at the basket from this position. He may also play with his back to the basket and use pivot and use pivot and hook shots from this position.

The third type of single post offense is one that is used by some teams in which utilization is made of a high post man. This player usually stations himself somewhere along the free throw line with his back to the basket. This type of post man is generally used more as a screener, feeder, and post than as a scorer. When he does make a scoring attempt, he must either turn and face the basket, or he must attempt to drive around his man toward the basket in order to make use of a close jump or hook shot. In his initial position he is usually too far away from the basket to be able to score effectively with his back to the basket. Therefore, the team using this type of offense generally makes use of more cuts and double cuts than used in the other types of single post offenses mentioned earlier.

DOUBLE POST OFFENSES

Sometimes a coach is fortunate enough to have more than one talented post player. He may want to make use of both players in the lineup at the same time. If neither of the players can make an adequate adjustment to the playing of a forward or wing position, then the coach will have to introduce the use of a double post offense. There are basically two types of double post offenses. One is what has traditionally been called the double post offense, and the other is the tandem post or 1-3-1 offense.

The team using a double post offense has two post men playing positions on either side of the foul lane. These post men may play in low post positions, but generally they play in medium high post positions. The other three players are placed in outside positions, generally one is a point man and the other two play the wing positions. The use of three out-double post style involves weaving maneuvers being made by the three outside players and then they in turn make double cuts off the pivot players. It is usually necessary that the point man be a capable ball handler since he is almost solely responsible for advancing the ball and initiating the offensive moves made by the team. The wing men are generally good outside shooters who also have enough speed to drive for the basket when the occasion presents itself. The post players usually screen for one another and execute driving pivot and turn around jump shots.

The tandem post (1-3-1) offense is generally utilized by a team when it has two post men in the starting lineup who have entirely different abilities. For example, one might be a taller player who is usually adept at scoring close to the basket, while the other might be much more mobile, but not necessarily a good scorer. At least one of the two players must be a good scorer. The high post in the tandem, like the high post in the single post offense, is used primarily as a feeder and screener. However, it is necessary that he is able to be an offensive threat from his position particularly with the use of a turn around jump shot. The low post in the tandem is usually a roving baseline player who may play very well with his back to the basket, or he may move further out along the baseline and face the basket for his shots. The three outside men generally need the same capabilities and perform the same movements as do those who play in the double post offense.

CONTINUITY OFFENSES

A team using the continuity offense is one that has its players always in motion and one that needs to do very little adjustment to "set it up" after retaining the ball on a missed shot at the basket. The Shuffle offense is an example of a continuity offense (see appendix). To play effectively with the use of a continuity offense a team must possess players with better than average mobility. Most teams that utilize such an offense also have players who are fairly equal in height. By their very nature, the use of continuity offenses does not result in a team getting as many attempts to score as would be true in the use of more free-lance types of offensive formations. In the continuity offense a team uses a particular sequence of screens and cuts so as to free its players for fairly high percentage shots. These maneuvers take time, and, therefore, the use of continuity offenses tends to "slow down" the play. Thus, it is not surprising to note that many of the college and university teams that annually lead statistically in defense employ continuity offenses. The amount of scoring done against such teams is often a reflection of the fact that they use a continuity offense rather than a reflection of their defensive prowess. The team using a continuity offense must have players who are good ball handlers, precise screeners, and, above all are mentally self-discipliners. If a team has these things, then the use of the continuity offense is highly recommended. It would be a most formidable task for any defense to try to stop them. It is not surprising then that many teams resort to the use of zone defenses to try to stop effectively teams that utilize the continuity offense.

FIVE MAN OUTSIDE OFFENSES

The advent of the tall, high scoring post man has tended to virtually eliminate the use of the five man outside offense. This type of offense involves the use of five players assembled in a spread formation, almost resembling that of a semi-circle, in the offensive area of the court. The use of such a formation lends itself particularly well to employment of three distinct types of offensive maneuvers. The first is utilization of the outside weave in which three, four, or all five of the players may be involved. The second is the use of a "flash" post where a player breaking from one of the outside positions into a post position, waits momentarily to receive a pass, and then if he does not receive the ball, moves back to one of the outside positions. The third is the "give and go" type of movement that was so popular in basketball a few years ago and is still utilized a great deal in the professional leagues today. All three of these maneuvers are difficult to defend against, and all three are effective if the proper type of player is available. Each player in the execution of these maneuvers must be able to move fairly quickly and each player must be able to dribble and handle the ball exceptionally well. If one or two of the players on the team does not possess these qualities, then the defense can easily sag off of their assigned men and effectively stop such offensive maneuvers made by the other players on the team. On the other hand, if the defensive team possesses one or two tall players who are not agile enough to effectively guard a man some distance away from the basket, then the use of the five man outside offense has a distinct advantage. In this latter case, the defensive team may be forced to go to the use of a zone defense to contain the players of the offensive team.

OFFENSES AGAINST ZONES

It has already been suggested that the basic team offensive style of play used against a man-to-man defense should be adaptable enough to be used also against a zone defense. Adherence to this principle will save the coach the time and effort he and his players would have to expend in teaching two different types of offenses to his players. Also, with the use of such an offensive pattern, the defensive team would be prevented from confusing the offensive team with a "cue" defense. (See section of team defense where discussion of the cue defense is presented, p. 166.)

There are several characteristics that each zone offense ought to possess.

(From here on zone offense shall be considered to mean the adaptation made of a regular, normal man-to-man offense that is also used against a team using a zone defense.) One such characteristic is continuous movement of all players. In today's game, it is almost mandatory that the players using offenses against zone defenses be in almost continuous motion. With the growing use of "flexing" zone defenses, the players using a zone offense where they just move to one position and stay in a certain area of the floor during the offensive phases of play will usually have little success. Also, this continuous movement should be constantly toward those parts of the zone defense that are most vulnerable.

Another characteristic involved with the use of the zone offense is that the players who are the best outside shooters try to be free to attempt the majority of shots taken at the basket. It is foolish for the team using the zone offense to have effective movement and sharp passing only to end up having the poorest shooter on the team take the shot at the basket. It is almost always necessary for a team to have to "shoot a team out of a zone defense." Therefore the better outside shooters should be allowed to have the opportunity to make the most attempts at the basket.

Another characteristic of the effective use of the zone offense is that the team using it attempts to penetrate the zone defense especially in the medium high or high post areas. Any team that can consistently pass the ball into the high post position will probably have success shooting against the zone defense. This is true for two reasons; first, the high post man often can attempt very good shots at the basket against a zone defense. Second, passes made by the high post player to other offensive players usually result in these players having the opportunity to take good shots because of their farther penetration of the zone defense toward the basket. This is because the players using the zone defense tend to "collapse" toward the center of the court to guard the high post man who has received the ball. When they do make the collapsing move, it momentarily frees other offensive players so that they can move closer to the basket in an attempt to take good shots at the basket.

While it is generally accepted as good policy to adapt the movement in the team man-to-man offense to create a zone offense, there is another procedure that is commonly used and may be considered to be acceptable in certain situations. Some coaches prefer to have their players move the ball quickly while remaining in set positions themselves. For example, against a 2-1-2 zone defense the offensive players may set themselves in a 1-3-1 alignment and remain in those positions. They then move the ball with sharp, quick passes and attempt to create a situation whereby the high percentage shot is taken. The drawback to the use of this method, of course, is the possibility of running into a team that plays a match-up type of zone defense. If in scouting, however, the opponents are found to play one type of zone defense without any flexing or matching-up, then the coach may want to utilize quick movements of the ball rather than having his players move in a pattern style or play.

This brief summary of basic offensive types is presented here to acquaint the reader with the wide range of possibilities the coach has in selecting an offensive formation for use by his team. The reader is encouraged to consult the appendix for a more detailed, diagrammatic presentation of many more offensive formation.

FAST BREAK OFFENSES

Many teams prefer to minimize the nature of the set offense in the opponent's forecourt while emphasizing the fast break. Fast break basketball can be very exciting to play and to watch, but it is very difficult to master. Fast break basketball can be played in combination with any of the offenses mentioned in this section, or it can be used in combination with a free-lance type of offense if the fast break does not eventuate. Many teams that utilize the fast break prefer to use a "pick-and-roll" offense once they set up in the opponent's forecourt. The pick-and-roll offense is quite simply the use of two against two offensive maneuvers anywhere in the opponent's forecourt. The pick-and-roll can be done between two guards, a guard and a forward, a guard and the center, or a forward and the center. It involves a screen, the dribbler moving by the screen, an attempt to force a switch by the defense, and a roll by the screener to the basket for a possible pass from the dribbler.

The fast break is practiced at times by almost every team regardless of the offensive formation used by them. However, to play fast break basketball the team must practice frequently the skills involved in such a maneuver. There are several key elements composing the fast break offense. First, a good defense helps make a fast break team. A good defense forces bad shots and usually results in a lower shooting percentage being made by the opponents. A lower shooting percentage means more missed shots, and every missed shot is an opportunity for a defensive team to have a fast break.

The second key element in the fast break is rebounding. A team cannot fast break until they secure the ball on the rebound. The section on rebounding should be consulted for principles and strategies associated with that phase of the game.

The third key element in the fast break is the outlet pass. This must be a quick, hard pass that travels as far upcourt as possible. Most successful fast break teams have one or more players who rebound well and are skilled at making the outlet pass. Contrary to popular belief, this kind of skill can be taught to most players. The two-hand overhand pass, the hook pass, or the baseball pass can all be utilized in the fast break outlet pass. The section on passing should be consulted for information on skills associated with this phase of the fast break.

It is generally felt that a neat three-man fast break should occur by having the outlet pass made to a player on the side court, a pass then made from the side court man to the middle-man, and then the rush up court by the player. In this way three lanes are created, filled by a middle-man and a man on each wing. This type of three-lane break is optimal and should be worked on at some length. However, fast breaks do not always occur as they are diagrammed on chalkboards. Lanes do not always get filled at precisely the right moment, and often there are two players rushing down court with a third man trailing. The point is that all such possible situations need to be practiced in order to build a successful fast break offense. General principles for passing and shooting should be evolved, but players will be successful in combatting the changing situations in a game only when they have encountered and learned about a sufficient number of different situations in practice. In this way they come to know how to react and to know how their own teammates react.

A two-man fast break often occurs and is very often badly played by the offensive team. Two men rushing down court on a break should not run on either side of the mid-line of the court. One player should establish control of the ball in the center lane while the other player fills a wing. It is much more difficult for a defender to play against a two man break when the middle and wing lanes are filled. This is because the defender, in order to stay between the two players, must move away from the center of the court.

The most common mistake made by players during fast break maneuvers is to maintain the dribble too long before passing. There are two distinct reasons why the player controlling the ball with the dribble should make a pass to a teammate by the time he reaches the area of the foul circle. First, the closer to the basket offensive players get, the easier it becomes for the defensive player to contain them. For example, the closer two offensive players get to the basket on a two-man break, the easier it is for one defender to thwart their efforts. Likewise, it is easier for two defenders to play against a three-man break if the dribbler keeps the ball until he reaches the foul line. The early pass makes the defender or defenders commit themselves and gets them moving. Once movement in the defense occurs, it is easier to create favorable offensive situations. A second reason for passing early is the speed at which players move on a well-executed fast break. A wing man running full speed on a fast break needs time to receive a pass and make his lay-up or short jump shot. If the dribbler keeps the ball too long, the wing man will either be too far under the basket to make a good shot or he will have to slow up, thus losing the step advantage he might have on a defender.

The fast break type of offense can be used after the opponents have made a basket or free throw. Getting the ball in bounds quickly and up the court quickly can create the same kind of momentary advantage that fast break teams strive for after starting a break for a rebounded shot. The same principles apply to fast breaks from inbounds passes as for breaks initiated from rebounded shots. Finally, an intercepted pass may bring about favorable fast break possibilities.

Team Defenses

It is generally true historically that defensive maneuvers used in basketball have developed in order to counter offensive procedures developed by both the individual player and the team. Another point to bear in mind in the study of basketball defense is that in the individual development of each player, the offensive skills of dribbling, passing, and shooting are learned long before the defensive skills. Team defenses in basketball then have generally developed as reactions to and follow in the wake of innovations developed by the offense. Thus, defenses have had to change and adapt to combat the increased offensive potential created by such innovations as the one-hand set shot, the jump shot, and the increased utilization of tall men in the post. If one would want to predict what defensive skills will be needed in the future, the most important factor to consider would be the prediction of what offensive skills will be developed. Likewise, the many and varied skills possessed by the offensive players in today's game of basketball require that defenses be flexible and adaptable, and that team defenses be truly a blending of the defensive skills of five players working in harmony with each other.

Defense in basketball has evolved from a man to man concept, in which the individual defensive player had responsibility for one man only, to the current concept of total team defense as mentioned above in which each individual player normally accepts responsibility for his own assignment and also that of aiding and abetting his teammates. Zone defenses, switching man-to-man defenses, pressing defenses, sagging defenses, and all the many in-between combination defenses stress having a blend of individual responsibilities and team defensive efforts in which the whole is greater than any of the component parts. The approach taken in this text is not one of heralding the value of any particular defense as a "best" defense, but rather to present principles, the use of which will allow the coach to choose that defense which best meets his immediate defensive needs, and to encourage the selection of that defense which is adaptable for use in many situations.

PRINCIPLES FOR SELECTING AND BUILDING EFFECTIVE TEAM DEFENSE

1. A defense should be selected on the basis of information secured from three primary sources:
   a. the characteristics of the players composing the home team,
   b. the characteristics of the players of the opposing team(s) and their composite as a team,
   c. the possible interactions that may take place between the home team and the opponents.
2. One defense should be selected and fully mastered as the primary defense.
3. However, all possible alternate defenses that might be used during a season should be practiced by the team during the preseason workouts.
4. Successful execution of a defense by a team requires that constant communication exists among the five defenders.
5. Team pursuit is the underlying strength of any team defense.
6. The coach must be much more concerned with his players' motivation and attitude when they are on defense than when they are on offense.

There are several factors that may influence the coach when he is developing the team defense. However, one must never forget that the coach does not enter into this decision making process with complete objectivity. The coach is a product of his previous playing and coaching experiences, and these may unduly influence him. If the coach has had experience with only man-to-man defenses while he was a college player, then he probably would not select a zone defense as the primary defense to use during his first year as a coach. This would probably be a wise decision. On the other hand, the experienced coach may have a more varied background and may be more adaptable in his selection. Yet he may have had great success with a zone defense thus he might be hesitant in switching from a zone to a man-to-man defense. Thus it is true that one is usually more adept at teaching that which one has had experience with than the reverse.

Another factor to consider in selecting a defensive formation is the quality and quantity of the team members. This information will weigh most heavily in determining the final decision. Listed below are questions about *his players,* the answers to which the coach should make before a final decision about the selection of a team defense is made. These include factors other than those above that must be considered in the selection.

The Home Team

HOW TALL IS THE FRONT LINE OF HIS TEAM?

If the front line (players who normally perform on offense near the basket) is tall and slow, a zone may be the most effective defense to use. However, if these players are tall and quick, the coach is virtually free to make a selection of any defense. The tall front line (provided the players are quick in their movements) can cover up for defensive mistakes made in the outcourt area thus making driving lay-ups very difficult to execute. Consequently, the guards (outside players) may play more aggressively than they might otherwise do. On the other hand, the tall front line players may not want to give up potential rebounding position by being too aggressive in their play. In this case, the short players in the front line will usually want to be very aggressive, regardless of how quick they are. However, having short front line players will cause a coach to want them to apply defensive pressure on their opponents at a distance that is as far away from the basket as possible. For example, if the short forward allows his man to receive the ball close to the basket he generally cannot stop him from shooting (he will go right over the top of him) at the basket. It is thus clear that the size and speed of the offensive players must be considered when the defensive formation is determined.

ARE THERE ANY QUICK, OUTSTANDING DEFENSIVE PLAYERS ON HIS TEAM?

The presence of one or two outstanding defensive players on the squad who are quick may warrant the choice of a defense that will make the best use of his or their abilities even though the rest of the team may not be very well suited to play the particular defense selected. This is especially true if these players are guards and are outstanding on defense. If these players are freed to be aggressive ball-hawks, they can change the entire complexion of a game. The number of men that the coach has that possess such special defensive traits or characteristics will help influence the coach in choosing a defense. Usually good players can play any type of defense. Limitations in player abilities limit the choices a coach has in selecting a team defense. When one or two players exhibit great defensive skill, the coach may want to use a combination defense that will enable them to utilize their skills without demanding more from the rest of the members of the team than they are able to perform.

HOW POOR ARE HIS WORST DEFENSIVE PLAYERS?

The answer to this question will help in determining the defensive formation that will be used. Sometimes a good offensive player is so poor defensively that the coach is limited in his selection of defenses. Having big slow forwards makes it almost impossible for the team to utilize an effective man-to-man defense. Guards who lack quickness make it impossible for the team to play a full court pressing defense. The coach must decide how to best cover up for the defensive weakness of his players by employing the most effective team defense he can devise.

WHAT IS THE PREVIOUS EXPERIENCE OF THE PLAYERS?

This is an extremely important question for the coach to answer at any level. There is a great deal of support for the opinion that basic man-to-man defenses (see section on individual defense) must be mastered before any other defense can be introduced. On the other hand, the coach who inherits a team composed of players who have played primarily a zone defense for most of their playing experience may well be better off to stick with the zone defense for the period he has these players, because they are more familiar with it and have had more experience playing it. The coach should not depend upon verbal answers to ascertain the past experience of his players, rather he should experiment with having his players use different defenses in order to determine the degree of experience they have had. Three years of experience incorrectly playing man-to-man defense is of little value to players as every good coach knows.

HOW AGGRESSIVE ARE THE PLAYERS DEFENSIVELY?

Some players are naturally more aggressive than others and the coach makes a judgment based on his appraisal of this trait about the aggregate aggressiveness of his team. Armed with this information a decision is made about the type of defense he will use in a given season. For example, the continuous use of a collapsing zone defense is psychological suicide for the team that is naturally aggressive, on the other hand employment of an aggressively player switching man-to-man defense is ineffective when the players lack aggressiveness.

Players can become more aggressive in their play if the coach emphasizes aggressiveness, makes it clearly understood what he means by aggressive play, and rewards those players who perform in this manner.

HOW EFFECTIVE OFFENSIVELY IS THE TEAM?

The presence of an offensive superstar may cause the coach to shy away from the use of aggressive defenses in which fouling is a natural consequence. Also a high powered offensive team may be better off playing a containment type defense rather than a pressing defense, while, on the other hand, a good offensive team may be able to afford the mistakes that the use of an aggressive defense usually entails. The team that is not so offensively minded will have to be concerned more about its defense, and thus will have to depend more upon it for team success. These considerations have important implications for the amount of practice time that should be spent on team defense as opposed to team offense.

Another source of information for the coach to have is the defensive and offensive styles of play used by opponents that play against his team. This is important to know at the beginning of the season and it is also an important factor to consider in preparing for each game. At the outset of the season, the coach must decide if the majority of his opponents use any particular basic offensive style of play, and he must make use of this information when he determines the basic team defense his team will use. Also, in preparing for each game, the coach must decide how best to adapt his basic defensive formation in order to combat the opponents style. Below are found some questions and statements about *opposing teams* which the coach should answer or consider regarding his opponent's style of offensive play before he decides on the type of defense he will have his team employ.

The Opponents

TO WHAT EXTENT DO THE OPPONENTS MAKE USE OF THE FAST BREAK?

If the opponents fast break a great deal, then a quickly retreating defense might be most effective to use in such a situation. If the opponents refuse to fast break under any conditions, then a pressing defense might be more successfully utilized, especially if the coach wants to speed up the game. If the coach has a strong rebounding team, then the fast break used by the opponents presents less of a defensive problem, but if his team is likely to be consistently out-rebounded, then the threat of the fast break being successful looms large.

WILL THE TEAM FACE A PREDOMINATELY CONTROLLED OR A FREE LANCE STYLE OF OFFENSE?

The controlled offense team often has as its goal opening lanes for its members to drive to the basket. The use of this type of offense might be best countered with a zone that will force the opponents to try the outside shot. On the other hand, a free lance offensively minded team often looks for and desires to take the good outside shot. This type of offense might be best countered by the use of an aggressive man-to-man defense that usually permits the offensive team to have an occasional drive to the basket in favor of preventing the good outside shot. The shuffle offense is particularly hard to defend against with the use of a man-to-man defense unless the defensive players are quite capable defensively. The team that relies on the big center for their scoring punch might be effectively stopped with the use of a sagging man-to-man or by employing a collapsing zone defense. The free lance offense style of play often makes use of the pick and roll feature as a part of its basic offense. A switching man-to-man, rather than a straight man-to-man, might be most effective to use against this offensive maneuver.

DO ONE OR MORE OF THE OPPOSING TEAMS HAVE ONE OR TWO WEAK SHOOTERS?

The presence of a weak shooter on the opposing team can allow the home coach to free one defensive player for part-time duty helping out where he is needed the most. For example, he might sag off on a big center. He might double team on a high-scoring forward. He might execute a trap maneuver on an offensive guard. He might sag into the open lane to pick up any offensive player driving toward the basket. This releasing of a player may prove to be a real asset to the team defensive effectiveness regardless of where a coach chooses to utilize it, and it is one that is not often enough explored for its possible use.

CAN THE OPPONENTS OFFENSE BE STOPPED AT ONE CRUCIAL POINT?

If an offense is initiated by a pass being made down the side of the court to a forward, the entire offense might be upset if the initial passing lane was consistently blocked by an aggressive defensive forward. If one guard acts as a "quarterback" for the entire offense, double teaming this guard on occasion might also be a useful strategy, especially if the guard is not too tall and would have difficulty passing out of a trap situation. Some offenses are unimaginative in the ways in which they react to this type of defensive pressure, and many games have been won by concentrating defensive pressure at a crucial point during an offensive maneuver, especially at a point at which the offense is being initiated.

THE RELATIVE COMPARISON OF TEAM CHARACTERISTICS

The third source of information, that of the interaction between teams, has already been briefly considered, but ultimately this becomes the only really meaningful source of information on which to plan the defensive strategy. The coach does not look at his own team or his team's opponent in an abstract manner. The characteristics which each team displays are therefore relative in nature. For example, he considers how tall is a front offensive line that averages 6 feet 4 inches in comparison to his team members. How fast are the guards? These questions take on significant meaning only when comparisons are made between the opposing team members. If the opponent's front line averages 6 feet 7 inches, then a 6 foot 4 inch defensive front line is not very tall. Decisions about selecting a team defense can be influenced by information about the relative characteristics of one team in comparison to another. If two teams are exactly equal in size, speed, etc., then the coach may choose virtually any defense he wants to use against his opponents. The more the teams differ, the more limited or expanded the coach's decision will become. Below are listed some of the more common differences found among teams and the defensive possibilities that may be employed in the given situations.

THE OPPONENTS ARE TALLER BUT NOT AS QUICK

This situation often occurs and the proper counter requires that an aggressive man-to-man or even a pressing defense of some type be utilized. The key deciding factor revolves around the attempt to assert the strengths of a team's defensive characteristics before the opponents get into that part of the court where their strengths will dominate the play. This suggests that defensive pressure be applied outside of the prime scoring area, and the play is thus shifted to that area of the court where quickness is a more important factor than height.

THE OPPONENTS ARE BETTER SHOOTERS

The key to employing successful defense in this situation is to make it as difficult as possible for the opponents to get good shots in those areas from which they prefer to shoot. This might be accomplished by an aggressive, pressing defense that applied pressure before the opponents reach the prime scoring area. It also might be accomplished by adapting a zone or man-to-man defense to apply maximum pressure in certain floor areas in the prime scoring area. For example, an opposing team that has two good forwards who shoot very well from the wing positions might be most effectively stopped by using a 1-3-1 zone defense that is very strong in the wing positions. Naturally, this will create weaknesses in other areas, but the point is that the opponent's favorite shooting area has been effectively taken away from them and they are forced to concentrate their shooting efforts from less familiar floor areas.

THE OPPONENTS ARE QUICKER BUT DO NOT SHOOT AS WELL

This almost always calls for the use of a defense that seals off the driving lanes, especially those toward the middle line of the lengthwise portion of the court. A sagging man-to-man defense may accomplish this as well as the use of many of the zone types, especially the 1-3-1 and 1-2-2 zones. The object here is to force the opponents to attempt the outside shot and to take away the driving shot where their quickness would give them a real advantage.

THE OPPONENTS ARE MUCH MORE DELIBERATE IN OFFENSIVE STYLE

In this situation, the coach must make the basic decision about what efforts he will have his team make to control the tempo of the game. He must either accept the slow tempo that the opponents prefer and let his team play this style, or he must have his team do something defensively in an attempt to speed up the tempo. The most common method used to speed up the tempo is the use of the full court pressing defense, but this often does not apply enough defensive pressure where it is most badly needed. Deliberate teams are often deliberate only in the offensive scoring area and this is where they should be pressured to speed up their play. Unfortunately, a full court pressing defense puts the most pressure on an offense in the back court. A pressing half-court defense or a trapping defense therefore would seem to be the best choices to use to achieve this goal. Each tends to force the deliberate team out of its normal pattern. As a consequence the defensive team is given offensive opportunities that must be taken advantage of or the use of the aggressive defense will take its toll.

There are, of course, many individual and team characteristics, interactions, and playing situations that have not been considered in selecting a team defense. It may serve the reader well to compile a much more exhaustive list of such information before deciding on the most effective team defense to use. However, the important concept that the reader should grasp from this discussion is that there are three primary sources of information, and that the information gained from these sources will probably be 90 per cent influential in the decision making concerning the selection of a team defense.

Whatever the choice, at least one defensive system should be selected by the coach and mastered as well as possible by the members of the team. It is no doubt true that a given coach is better suited in terms of personality and experience to coach one type of defense over another type of defense. Nevertheless, at least one type of defense should be adequately learned if the team is to be successful. While it is relatively easy individually to learn the skills and techniques of defensive play, it takes a great deal of practice for a team as a unit to master a defensive system, and to be able to adapt it effectively to various game situations. Also, it is questionable whether a young team can master more than two defenses in any given season unless the team members have had a great deal of previous experience. The coach might want to select a basic man-to-man and a basic zone defense and have his team become proficient in the use of these two defensive procedures. The key to mastering a defensive system so that it will be functional in the game situation is to subject the players to enough practice under varying conditions so that the team will learn to adapt effectively their basic defensive moves to many and varied conditions. A serious mistake that is often made by a coach is to have the first team work only against the same defense as their own in practice sessions. In team defensive practice, it is believed that it is better to have the offensive unit use many type of offenses, especially those which the coach knows his team will face during the season.

There are situations when the coach will feel justified in having his team utilize a defense that is not one of the basic team defenses he has selected for use during the season. For example, he may want to employ a zone with a chaser for one game only in an attempt to stop a hot shooter on the opponent's team. He may also want to use a full court press as a surprise tactic for one game only. The defenses that a coach might use, that he does not consider as part of his basic defensive repertoire for the team to normally use, should be practiced during the early pre-season sessions. Especially those defenses that the coach has in the past used only on occasion should be practiced by the team at this time. One such early practice session spent on learning the zone and chaser defensive formation may prove to be immensely beneficial at a later time in the season when the coach decides that the zone and chaser would be a good surprise tactic to use for a particular game. The team will then not be totally unfamiliar with the defense and how to play it. Also, the players will be able to pick up the fundamental concepts involved in the use of the defense much more easily in this recall situation. This would be an easier learning situation than if they were confronted with practicing the defense procedure for the first time. It would probably be very beneficial if the team could, in their early practice sessions, become familiar with the fundamentals of one pressing defense, a defense to counter a stalling attack, a preventative defense to guard against excessive fouling, a defense to stop one very hot scorer, a defense to use against a fast break, and a defense to use against a tall center.

Communication among the defensive players is often the difference between the execution of an excellent team defense and one in which the players make a few too many errors to be effective. This is especially true when the man-to-man varieties of the team defenses are used. When defense evolved from the individual concept to the team concept, communication became a vital part of the total team defense. Communication means verbal exchange between and among players unless the coach is fortunate enough to have five mystics on the floor, all of whom possess extrasensory perception. Unfortunately, some players perform as if they expected their teammates to have ESP, that is they think of the team making the right move, but do not verbally communicate this to their teammates. The result is that too often a basket is scored by the opponents because of lack of communication. Why basketball players are so prone to be silent on defense is one of the great mysteries of the game, but it is a problem that must be solved if the team defense used is to be successful. For example, in a switching man-to-man defense, communication is probably the most important part of the defense. The responsibility lies with the defender guarding the screener to alert the defender guarding the player with the ball that a screen may be impending and from which direction the screen is coming. Then, the defender guarding the screener must make the decision as to whether a switch is necessary. If so, he must verbally communicate this fact so that there can be no doubt that his teammate has heard him. The language of the call is more important than it is often considered to be. It may be stated that one patterns himself to react to a certain verbal cue so that his actions become virtually automatic in nature, but still dependent on a certain cue to trigger off their execution. The more cues that are used to elicit the response, the more difficult and slow the learning of the proper response will become. In a switch situation the defender may yell "I've got him," "I'll take him," "mine," "switch," or any other of a number of verbal cues. However, the most important point to remember is that the coach must choose one verbal signal. All of the players must adhere to the use of that signal in switching situations. Dedication to this principle will lessen the confusion that too often occurs when using a switching man-to-man defense.

Switching is certainly not the only situation in which communication between and among players is not only desirable but necessary. Whenever a player has his back to a teammate, verbal communication is the best means available to be sure that the two players will work together and not independently. The use of a sagging defense to protect against a big pivot man or to cut off driving lanes requires a great deal of communication so that each lane is filled at the right moment. A trapping or pressing defense requires communication so that the crucial trapping moment will be taken full advantage of by the players involved.

Football coaches spend a great deal of their defensive practice time working on pursuit, and it would serve basketball coaches well to ponder this idea and put it into use. Webster defines pursuit as "following in order to overtake; to continue to annoy or distress." This definition serves very well the sports concept of pursuit. In football, pursuit means to select the right angle to cut off a player and stop him at a certain location. In basketball it can mean virtually the same thing. Whether a zone, man-to-man, a pressing or sagging defense is used, pursuit is often the difference between team success or failure. There are two aspects to remember in the teaching of pursuit. First, pursuit must become a state of mind so that the proper thing is done in any given situation. That is, the player must become so convinced that pursuit is part of his defensive assignment that he reacts as a matter of automatic response. Second, the coach must make players aware of their own speed, the speed of opponents, and the angles that must be taken to pursue and cutoff an opponent effectively. To simply follow after an opponent will not get the job done, but to pursue him at an advantageous angle and cut him off will add immeasurably to the defensive effectiveness of the team.

Coaches must remember that they will have to be more concerned with motivation and attitude in teaching defense than they will in teaching offense. Most coaches find that they have to provide very little motivation to get a player to work diligently on offense, yet often the coaches on the other hand have to supply a great deal of motivation for a player to enjoy defense. To have his team be successful defensively, the coach must instill an attitude within the players that is conducive to successful execution of the defense. There are four aspects of this problem that merit discussion and may serve as guidelines toward successful solution of this problem.

First, the coach must instill an offensive attitude in the defensive players. That is, the team must play defense, but not play it defensively, but rather play it as if it were merely an extension of the offense that will help win the game for them. A defense cannot be timid. It must assert itself, indeed, it must "offend" the opponents. It may be easier for the coach to instill this type of attitude in his players if he uses an aggressive defense than if he employs a so-called non-aggressive defense such as a conventional zone. (This does not mean that the occasional use of a non-aggressive defense would not be enjoyed by the players as a surprise tactic.) It is possible to instill this offensive attitude into a team using any defense and the so-called non-aggressive defenses can be very aggressively executed and consequently much more effective.

The second and third aspects of this problem are closely related to each other and should be considered together. The idea that defense is a difficult job that must be done is not terribly conducive to consistently successful defensive play. Players have to believe that playing defense is challenging and rewarding, and therefore fun to do. In order to get players to exhibit this attitude they must be rewarded for a job well done. When a player does his job well on offense, he most often is tangibly rewarded by having the ball go through the basket. The fans see this and they respond to it. However, the coach (often alone) must reward successful defensive play by giving recognition of some sort to the players. It matters little to this discussion what that recognition is, but players who are rewarded for their defensive efforts will easily develop the attitude that defense is fun to play, and when that moment comes the player will no doubt, within the limits of his ability, become a very proficient defensive player.

The fourth aspect of the problem of motivation and attitude on defense is the question of responsibility. Many coaches believe that using a straight man-to-man defense is the only way to determine properly defensive responsibility. We do not agree with this concept. Coaches, players, and even many fans know when a player has fallen down on his defensive responsibility regardless of the defense that is being used. When opponents are scoring consistently from one side of a zone, someone in the zone defense can be held responsible. When a pressing defense is being broken consistently either by passing or dribbling, defensive responsibility is not difficult to pinpoint. Players must be made to realize that their responsibility might be either to a man, to a territory or an area on the floor, or to a situation, but that they do have a responsibility and will be held accountable for carrying out their responsibility. However, it must be kept in mind that team defense means all members of a team helping each other. Sometimes an opposing player is just too good on offensive for one man to stop him alone. Help is needed so more than one man may at times guard one opponent for a brief time.

Various Defensive Systems

MAN-TO-MAN TEAM DEFENSES

There are several basic decisions that have to be made before a coach decides to use a man-to-man defense. The most important of these decisions is concerned with how each individual will play his assigned man. Most coaches like to establish a pattern of playing individual man-to-man defense within the total team context. There are several possibilities that might be used in the relation to this concept: (1) head-on or "honest" defense, (2) overplaying to the outside, (3) overplaying to the inside, (4) overplaying to either the non-preferred or preferred hand side of the offensive player, and (5) playing loosely or closely and/or aggressively. Each of these alternatives has a different purpose, but the important point here is that a man-to-man team defense may be made much more effective if all five players understand their own and each other's assignments. The better the opponents, the more honest the man-to-man defense must be. Most coaches would prefer to force the offense to the inside because this is where additional defensive help is most readily available. Others prefer to have their players force the right-handed player to go to his left, assuming that he will be much less of an offensive threat in that direction. Finally, some prefer to have their defensive players as a team play a loose man-to-man defense, a constantly aggressive man-to-man, a tight man-to-man, or a man-to-man whereby the degree of pressure is varied according to the situation.

Also, another basic team decision that the coach will have to make involves the question of how switching will be accomplished. The players using a man-to-man defense must at some time or other resort to the switch. Some teams will want to switch at the occurrence of every screen as a matter of policy. The coach will have to decide how he wants his players to execute the switch. Communication has already been cited as a key factor in determining the effectiveness of the switch. When the coach has decided when he wants his players to switch, he will then have to decide, again as a matter of team policy, how he wants the switch to be executed. In summary then when to switch, what communication to use during the switch, and how to execute the switch seem to be three team considerations that must be accomplished.

THE STANDARD OR STRAIGHT MAN-TO-MAN DEFENSE

The players using this defense will switch only when it is absolutely necessary. The players attempt to stay with their assigned men unless they are definitely screened out of the play. The coach using this defense finds it relatively easy to fix individual responsibility. This can be a strong motivating factor in encouraging the players to put forth great effort. However, this defense is most difficult to use against offenses which involve a great deal of player movement and make use of numerous screens such as that found in the Shuffle offense. It will probably be most effective to use against teams that employ a basic pattern style of play with provisions made for a great deal of free lancing. When a player desires to stay with his man, there are three routes he may take to get by a screen and remain with his assigned opponent. He may go over the top of the screen, that is he may try to "beat" the screen: he may slide through the gap between the screener and his defensive teammate; or he may go behind the screen and his defensive teammate. The degree of aggressiveness that the coach wants to have his players display will probably determine his policy in this connection. Generally speaking, the sliding through method will be the most successful to use in most cases. The attempt to "beat" the screen will be the movement utilized by the very aggressive team. The going behind the other two players method is usually used only as a last resort.

THE AGGRESSIVE MAN-TO-MAN DEFENSE

This defense may be used in either a switching man-to-man or a straight man-to-man, but regardless, it is executed aggressively, and this is the main characteristic of this type of man-to-man defense. If the players use a straight man-to-man, the defender will most often try to beat any screen that is set. If they use a switching man-to-man, the switch will be an aggressive one that attempts to cut off the dribbler from his intended path. The players using this defense will pick the guards up near the half-court line and will challenge passes made to teammates that players using a standard man-to-man defense would allow to occur unchallenged. This defense has been popular for use by teams that are outmanned in height, but not in quickness. It has also been used successfully against teams that are not particularly adept at ball handling and passing. This defense is used primarily as an "equalizer" by a team that might be outmanned if its players used a standard man-to-man defense.

THE SWITCHING MAN-TO-MAN DEFENSE

The players using this defense will switch almost automatically when any screens are used. In this sense they may well reassemble into a zone type defense on occasion. When switching is a matter of policy, the switch can be anticipated and executed smoothly and rapidly, thus preventing the quick jump shot from being executed for which so many screens are designed. The player guarding the screener will play high on the inside of his man because it is not his responsibility to worry about a reverse roll being made by his opponent toward the basket. Playing high on his opponent a player can then switch quickly and smoothly to the other offensive player moving off the screen. The player guarding the man who sets the screen will play his man tight until the screen is made. Then he will drop back quickly to cover the path behind the screener and his defensive teammate. He thus prevents the roll toward the basket from being made and a pass back being received by the offensive player. The switching man-to-man can be used effectively only if the players communicate well among themselves. Each must know when one or more players intends to switch. If this condition is met, then this can be a very effective defense to use against continuity offenses that make use of a great deal of screening. Since these offenses are based upon the effective use of the screen as a major offensive weapon, the switching man-to-man may, if executed properly, completely immobilize the offense and force the players to take bad shots or to make errors. The switching man-to-man is the most effective defense to use when there is not a great mismatch in the heights of the players. The main weakness in the use of this defense is that there is the possibility of the offensive players creating a situation where a small defender has to play against a tall offensive player close to the basket. If this occurs frequently, a different type of defense will have to be used.

THE SAGGING MAN-TO-MAN DEFENSE

This form of the man-to-man defense is characterized not by the defensive action occurring at the ball, but rather by the defensive movements made by the four players who are not immediately involved with the ball. These four players play according to a zone principle, that is, they sag to cover lanes between the man with the ball and the basket. This defense has been popular for use by many coaches because it tends to combine the strengths of the man-to-man and the zone defenses. Its major weakness lies in the fact that it is vulnerable to good outside shooting teams, just as any zone defense is. The sagging player may not be able to return to his man quickly enough to prevent him from attempting the quick, outside shot. Therefore, this defense is probably a good defense to use against any team except that team whose players' main offensive ability is good outside shooting. It is a particularly good defense to use against a team that combines good guard play with a high scoring center. The use of the man-to-man features will produce maximum coverage of the passing lanes into the post area.

THE TRAPPING MAN-TO-MAN DEFENSE

A trap occurs when two defensive players double team an offensive player who possesses the ball. This move usually occurs by design at some designated area on the floor, or at a designated point of action. The players using a trapping man-to-man defense may attempt to trap in one or many situations. Some coaches like to have their defensive guards trap the dribbler just as he crosses the center court line. The dribbler is especially vulnerable to a trap when he turns his back to the opposing guard(s). Thus the center line is used as an "extra sideline" in that passes can be thrown only upcourt once the guard has crossed the line into his offensive half of the court. Other coaches prefer to have their defensive players execute a trap whenever two offensive guards or a guard and a forward cross each other's path with the ball. Still others prefer to use the two corners at the end of the offensive half of the court as trapping areas. Some will have their players trap anywhere on the court when feasible. The players initiate the attempt by means of a verbal signal between certain teammates. This defense is by design an aggressive type of the man-to-man variety, and it is often used during the later stages of the game when a team is behind, yet when the defensive team does not care to resort to the full court or half court styles of press. This defense is played quite similarly to other types of man-to-man defenses until the trap is executed. Then the remaining three players on the defensive team play a zone attempting to cut off the potential passing lanes from the trapped player to his teammates. Several guidelines may be established for the proper execution of the trap. They are: (1) the trap is most effectively executed on an offensive player who no longer has the dribble option, (2) a good time to make use of the trap is when the dribbler turns his back to one of the defensive players. (3) the players using the trap should seal off the areas that are the ones in which the trapped player is most likely to pass, (4) the most effective trap occurs when both defensive players spread themselves apart on the court and use their hands to block the passing lanes rather than make an attempt to steal the ball, and finally (5) once an offensive player has been trapped he should never be fouled by the defensive player. Rather, he should be forced to make a bad pass or forced into a held ball situation.

Zone Defenses

As with the use of the man-to-man defense, there are several basic decisions that need to be made before deciding to use the zone defense. No zone defense can be equally effective against an outside and inside shooting team. The coach will have to decide if he is more concerned about stopping shots made from the offensive perimeter, or is he more concerned about stopping shots made from the lane or pivot area. The answer to this question, more than any other, will help determine his choice of a zone defense to use. Another item that will effect his choice is the rebounding power of his team and their opponents. Some zones are particularly designed to make use of defensive rebounding strength, while others are not. Another item to consider is that of aggressiveness. Players using a zone can play with varying degrees of aggressiveness. Aggressiveness by players using a zone can harass an offense just as much as aggressiveness in a man-to-man defense can do.

Much has been said and written about the maneuvers players should make in a zone defense. Certain standard team and individual players should make in a zone defense. Certain standard team and individual player movements have generally been agreed upon for use by most coaches. However, with a little imagination and insight, many combinations of movements can be developed for use in a zone which bring about basically the same results. It is best to explore several possible movements that might be made with the use of the chosen zone. The most moves possible should be given to those players who are the quickest and best able to cover a given territory. In this way the coach can take maximum advantage of his strong defensive players, and cover up for his weakest players. The application of this concept leads to lesser amounts of movement for the big men who may tire more easily, and who also should be stationed closest to the basket as defensive rebounders (where less territory to cover is available).

THE 2-3 OR 2-1-2 ZONE DEFENSE

This defensive formation is quite likely the most widely used zone in basketball. There is some thought that its widespread use may be due to the fact that it allows a team to have the best combination of inside and outside coverage of the opponent's offensive formations. The use of this zone is most effective against a team that has good outside shooting from the guards and strong scoring from the pivot area. It is also, most likely, the best zone to use for securing the best defensive rebounding positions. The team that uses this zone is probably weakest against teams that have good scoring forwards. This is because the players cannot cover the wing or corner positions effectively. They may choose to cover one of the two scoring players effectively or both of them in a rather inadequate manner. They cannot cover both of them well and still utilize a true 2-3 zone. Also in using this zone they may have problems covering the roving baseline players, and it is often this player that causes the downfall of the zone.

THE 3-2 ZONE DEFENSE

The 3-2 zone defense is not utilized very often, yet it is quite likely the strongest zone defense to use against the outside shooting of the offensive team. Conversely, it is probably the weakest of the zone defenses to use in covering the lane or pivot area. The team is also vulnerable to good shooting from a roving baseline player. Nevertheless, for defending against the guard and forward shooting from the center top of the key area, the wing, and the corner, this zone is the most effective to use. Another weakness in using this zone is that it causes the team to have a lack of rebounding power. Thus, the particular combination of factors mentioned makes this a good zone for a quick, aggressive team to utilize.

THE 1-2-2 ZONE DEFENSE

The 1-2-2 zone defense is another popular and widely used defense. The teams who use it are strong in covering the lane or pivot area, the baseline area, and are generally effective in defensive rebounding. The use of this zone is popular with coaches who have players with good over-all height. However, they believe that their players lack the quickness necessary to employ effectively a man-to-man defense. One glaring weakness of the use of this zone is the inability of the players to defend against corner shots. The team who uses it is also vulnerable to weakside rebounding, but this limitation can be overcome by having the two wing players crisscross as the ball is moved across court. Thus the larger back wingman is freed to rebound on the weakside. There is some feeling among many students of basketball that the 1-2-2 zone is the best to use in defending equally well to the inside and outside. This belief is based on the fact that it is more difficult (than in other zone formations) for an offensive team to cause a defensive team to come out of a 1-2-2 set up even though they are temporarily scoring effectively.

THE FLEXING OR MATCH-UP ZONE DEFENSE

The use of this zone defense has gained widespread popularity in recent years because it tends to prevent an offensive team from playing an immoble set alignment (non-player movement) against it. For example, many coaches will have their players go immediately into a 1-3-1 offensive alignment if they know that a 2-3 zone is being played against them. This zone formation is flexible enough so that a team may shift to the 1-3-1 defensive alignment to counter the offensive movement. The principle utilized in the flexing zone or match-up zone is that the defensive players appear to pick up the offensive players in a standard man-to-man defense, but really they intend to employ a zone in essence from that time on until a definite shift in offensive alignment has occurred and then they flex to counter the new alignment. The value of utilizing this zone is obvious as the team tends to defend in those areas in which there are offensive threats. This zone has no structural weakness, but it is extremely difficult to use effectively in all situations. It is a hazardous defense to use unless it is well executed. Improper execution of the flexing zone creates absolute confusion and mayhem on the floor and often makes it extremely easy for the offensive team to penetrate the defense. The proper use of this zone requires that the players have had a great deal of experience. Also, communication on the part of the players is a necessity.

THE PRESSING OR TRAPPING ZONE

This defense is much like the trapping man-to-man previously mentioned except that the formation originates out of a zone rather than from a man-to-man set up.

The traps, however, can be executed at the same situations as is done in the trapping man-to-man. Once a trap has been accomplished the two defensive setups appear to be virtually identical. Many coaches like to spread their players out to cover the full offensive half of the court utilizing this zone formation. Thus in principle they are using a half-court pressing zone. It can be played as a part of a 2-3, 3-2, 1-2-2, or 1-3-1 zone, but is more often used in connection with a 1-2-2 zone.

Combination Defenses

In recent years, many coaches have experimented with the use of combination defenses and found them to be highly satisfactory. The purpose of the combination defense is to get "the best of both," that is, the best features of the zone and the man-to-man defenses are used by the players. The flexing zone is sometimes considered to be a combination defense, although here it is treated as a zone defense. The flexing zone does help to point out the strengths and weaknesses of combination defenses in that its proper use depends primarily on execution rather than on structure for its success. The same may be said of combination defense. Combination defenses are difficult to use but if executed properly are often energetic and stalwart defenses. Any coach can create a combination defense for use by his players to meet his particular needs. Indeed, one of the primary strengths of combination defenses is its possible maximum use by strong defensive players, and perhaps it offers minimum difficulty in its utilization by the weaker defensive players. Listed here are several of the more popular types of combination defenses.

THE ZONE WITH A CHASER DEFENSE

The zone with a chaser defense is quite likely the oldest of the combination defenses. This defense is most often employed against the team who has a prolific scorer that must be stopped. However, coaches may do well to consider its use in other instances. The great strength of using such a zone, or any other combination on occasion, is that some teams seldom practice against this type of defense and therefore would be unfamiliar with it. This is especially true if the offensive team does not possess a high scorer. The team that has no outstanding scorer quite likely has not spent one single minute of practice time working against a zone with a chaser. The element of surprise will often upset an offensive team completely if confronted with such a defense. In design, the defensive team employs a four man zone, and frees one defensive player to guard closely the best scorer on the opponent's team. The four man zone players usually take a position on the floor that is box-like in appearance, but they may also form together in a four man diamond which is also quite effective.

THE TRUE COMBINATION DEFENSE

The players utilizing the true combination defense most often employ a zone along the back-line and a man-to-man defense out on the floor against the offensive guards. Depending on the offensive formation that they are pitted against, they may also be in a two man zone in the backline with the three outside defensive men playing man-to-man. They may also be in a three man zone with the two defensive guards playing man-to-man. Some coaches even prefer to divide the floor lengthwise instead of crosswise for defensive purposes. This means that the guard and forward on one side will play a zone, while the guard and forward on the other side will play man-to-man. Again it may be said that the successful use of these defenses depends on the execution rather than on the structure. More practice must be spent on perfecting the use of the combination defenses than is necessary with the more traditional types of defense.

CUE DEFENSES

A cue defense is not a combination of the features of the man-to-man and zone defenses molded into one overall defense. Rather, it is a changing defense whereby the players switch back and forth from a man-to-man to a zone defense depending upon the situation. The switching may be controlled by a predetermined plan, such as every third time down the floor the players change, or the alternating may be controlled by verbal cues from the coach or one of the players on the floor. The players in a cue defense usually employ alternately one of the standard zones and one of the more standard man-to-man types of defense. The key to the success of the use of a cue defense is that the players constantly communicate among each other. Needless to say, it will be slightly confusing if only one or two of the players receive the cue and respond to it and the other players do not. The defense may also be cued on offensive movements made by the opponents. When the offensive team employs more than one offensive formation during a game, the coach may want to use a different type of defense against each offense. In this case, the cue is given to them by the opponents when they change their offensive formations.

Full-Court or Pressing Defenses

Like combination defenses the use of full-court or pressing defenses has been popular in recent years. Particularly is this true by teams that like to fast break offensively and who desire to control the tempo of the game. The pressing defense often makes for a faster moving game and this is to the advantage of the fast breaking team. The techniques of the teams utilizing these defenses are radically different from those used in half-court defenses, except that the range of movement by the players is greatly increased. This, of course, makes it difficult for the team that lacks quickness to use a full-court defense effectively. Some of these defenses are mentioned below.

THE MAN-TO-MAN PRESSING DEFENSE

The man-to-man pressing defense may take on many appearances. The players using it may in fact be in any one of the several half-court man to man defenses that has been extended to be full-court in character. The players do not need to be in a trapping man-to-man defense although they will tend to do so the more aggressive they are in their play. If the coach wants his players to use the pressing man-to-man defense just to insure a fast tempo in their play, then this defense will be one of the standard variety and just enough pressure will be exerted against their opponents to develop the desired tempo. When the man-to-man press the players employ is basically a trapping man-to-man defense, it is played quite similarly as the half-court defense. The primary difference in the two is the place on the floor where the trap is attempted. Regardless, most coaches prefer that the trap be executed as close to the sideline as possible thus limiting the areas where a pass may be thrown.

THE ZONE PRESS

Not too many years ago it was believed that a team could not use a zone press against top flight competition. This belief prevailed because it was thought to be too vulnerable to a good passing team. Needless to say, this has completely vanished and those coaches that hesitated to make use of the zone press probably were quickly converted to its use once they had it successfully used against them. It is unlikely that any team today can go through the season without using the zone press or having it used against them. Zone presses are basically trapping zone defenses extended to a coverage of the full court. Again, it may be stated that the only basic difference between the full-court and half-court pressing defenses lies in the range of the players' movements. The two basic formations most often utilized are the 1-2-2 and the 1-2-1-1. The latter is often referred to as the "diamond and one" zone press. One thing that the coaches often differ on in the use of the zone press is in the placement of the quick guards. Some coaches prefer that their quicker players play in the front line of the trapping areas of the zone press. Others prefer to have taller forwards play in the front line or trapping area. They want their quicker players to play in the middle line where they can use their quickness in an attempt to intercept passes. It should be emphasized at this point that the main purpose in utilizing the zone press is to have the players try to intercept passes rather than to attempt to steal the ball from the dribbler. The idea is to have the players trap the dribbler and to force him to make a difficult pass which can be intercepted. Fouling the dribbler or the man in the trap is a cardinal sin when using this defense.

Strategy

Strategy here refers to the art and science of conducting a basketball campaign in which a coach manipulates and maneuvers his players within the rules as they play against their opponents. It involves immediate tactics as well as long range objectives. It refers to offensive and defensive choices made by the coach and players, as well as to many other facets of the game that might eventually affect its outcome. These are done to gain advantage over another team. The coach is a strategist as he prepares for upcoming games during practices, and he is a tactician when he makes spur-of-the-moment decisions in the midst of a heated contest. Strategy, then, may be thought of as game generalship.

Some coaches believe that the starting point for the effective use of strategy is during pre-game practice. For example, some coaches like to bring their teams on the floor very early before a game, while others prefer to wait until the opponents are already on the floor before they make their entrance. Then, they may begin to employ strategy during the pre-game workout. Participation in the pre-game drills should provide the players with adequate warm-up in both the physiological and neuro-muscular sense. They can also be utilized both to prepare the team psychologically for the upcoming contest, and to help intimidate the opponents. Some coaches believe that having their players perform very intricate and "fancy" drills will accomplish this. However, it is probably more correct to assume that it is the crispness, preciseness, and enthusiasm shown by the players during the drill workouts that gain the effect wanted rather than the participation in intricate and complicated drills. Another point concerning strategy is involved in the players the coach uses at any one time. Generally speaking, the coach should have in the game at any one moment the five players who best fit the situation at hand. Thus, the coach must utilize his player talent to fit the needs of the situation. It is doubtful that there are often five players who will be the five best players to use in all situations. Therefore, the coach may want to make one or possibly two changes in his regular lineup when his team is competing against a particular opponent. Also, he may want to do so during a game when the situation calls for a change in tactics. Thus, the coach may want occasionally to play his five best shooters, his five best defensive players, his five best pressers, or his five most aggressive players. The idea is that the coach must attempt to always have his five best players on the floor in accordance with the needs of the game at the moment.

The coach must plan some of his team's strategy on the basis of what he sees happening on the floor during the game. While he may have prepared a basic game plan, he must be ready and willing to change it to meet the needs created by the situation that occurs at any particular moment. The coach must be constantly aware of the potential weaknesses in the opponent's offense or defense styles, and when they appear he should be able to adapt his plans to take advantage of such faults. One of the greatest handicaps that a basketball coach has is that his view (from the bench at floor level) during the game is not from a particularly good vantage point for spotting overall strengths and weaknesses in the opponent's offense and defense. It might be helpful for the coach to station an assistant high up in the gymnasium (on the top row of the bleachers, for example) in order for him to receive more accurate information on the opponents. If the assistant sees any developments worthy of reporting he could come down at the quarter or halftime break (or more often) and converse with the head coach on these matters.

Some matters of general strategy can be decided on before the game begins. However, some of them may have to be changed during the game. Falling under this category of general strategy would be such matters as defensive assignments, when and how much the team should fast break, when to press, when to slow down the tempo of the game, and when to take time-outs. As a general rule, it is advantageous to conserve the number of time-outs used so that there are some left for use near the end of the game when the players are likely to be more fatigued. Also, strategic decisions are likely to be more crucial at that time as they may have more effect on the outcome of the game. Time-outs are needed for discussions of certain maneuvers that may be used at this time. It should be stressed that while most of these matters may be a part of the general team policy, they must be approached in a flexible manner so that they can be readily adapted to meet the exigencies of the game situation.

A large part of strategy in basketball is involved with the action taken by a team in the closing minutes of a tightly contested game. Perhaps the biggest question is when to press if a team is behind or when to stall if it is ahead. These questions cannot be answered categorically, and it is up to the individual coach to reach a decision on these matters often during a stressful situation. One principle that needs to be clearly stated here, however, is that the team needs to be subjected to a variety of circumstances in practice in order to be effective under such conditions in game situations. For example, if the coach believes that his team should always stall when it has a slight lead during the closing minutes of a game, then his team must incorporate the stall as part of their basic offensive pattern that they practice each week. It is unfortunate that coaches often expect their players to perform adequately in the stall or pressing situation when they have not been given ample opportunity to practice it. Consequently, they do not develop the skills necessary to master such tactics.

Another situation that occurs more often than coach's practice plans would seem to indicate is the end of the game circumstances in which the score is tied or just one or two points separate the two teams. The coach is then confronted with the following questions: Should the team take a good shot as soon as it is possible or should the players wait and attempt the last "one shot"? Who should take the last shot? These questions generally should be answered during practice time so that the situation is not a totally unfamiliar one to the players when it occurs during the game. A special play may be developed for use in such situations if the coach desires. However, this is not nearly as important as the need for the practice of experiencing the "last shot" emergency.

Unusual or different facilities than the team is used to may call for a change in game tactics. For example, it is known that a loose open net enables a team to retrieve the ball after a successful shot and pass it in from out of bounds sooner than if a tight net is used. This is an advantage to a fast breaking team. A tight backboard reduces the effectiveness of a good rebounder. A stage court often bothers the shooters on the side away from the crowd because the target area is less discernible than in a four-walled gymnasium court.

The Organization of Practice Sessions

The most important point to mention concerning practice sessions is that they ought to be effectively and highly organized. The head coach along with his assistants should make plans ahead of time that embrace the use of every minute of a session. This is not to say, however, that there can be no deviation from such a plan. But rather to state that it is best to have a detailed plan from which deviations can be made if a situation develops where more time is needed on one aspect over another. The organizational plan should also include information on what every player will do at each minute during the session. All players ought to be constantly involved in doing something during the entire session. There is no reason why some players should be sitting on the sidelines watching their teammates practicing vigorously unless they are there because they need to rest for a few moments. Players can practice floor shooting, free throwing, one-on-one offensive and defensive maneuvering and/or any other movements necessary to the successful acquisition of needed skills. They should not be just sitting and watching. The only possible exception to this might be if the coach wanted certain players to follow closely the action taking place on the floor in order that he might point out some errors and good moves to them. Even in this case, the players who are not directly connected with the action would be better off just moving up and down the sidelines in keeping up with the action, and practicing movements that they see taking place out on the floor than just sitting.

Practices should be fast and short rather than long and slow. It is often of special benefit to most players to have the practice tempo set to emulate the game tempo. Games are approximately one hour and forty-five minutes in length overall. Therefore, the practice session should be conducted at a fast paced tempo in line with the time allotted for a game. Long practices tend to take the edge off of performance, and this could be detrimental to motivation. Players can still learn while tired, but the coach should be very careful about practices that might damage player motivation even though some learning may still occur.

Early in the season the coach most likely will spend more time in developing offensive skills and perfecting a team offense than he does in developing defensive skills and a team defense. However, as the season progresses, this pattern might well be changed, as more and more practice time may be spent on practicing defensive maneuvers that will be utilized in the impending games. As was mentioned elsewhere, players need to spend more time in developing offensive skills than they do in developing defensive skills. Therefore, the early season practices may be scheduled so more time is devoted to the offense rather than the defense phases of the game.

The player must spend a great deal of time in practice on his shooting skills. For this reason, extra practice time may be scheduled for the perfection of these skills, but this time must be spent purposefully. If the coach allows his players to spend fifteen or twenty minutes before and after practice perfecting the shooting skills, he should make sure that the practice is conducted in a purposeful manner. The player should probably not be shooting alone. That is, he should do it under defensive harassment. Shooting at the basket by a player should also be done from only those parts of the floor where the players are most likely to take a shot during the game situation. Foul shooting is best practiced during the regular practice session and not after the formal session is over. The coach may have small, intermittent sessions of foul shooting interspersed with scrimmage. This allows the players to practice foul shooting when they are somewhat fatigued and is more similar to the game situation than any other procedure. It also prevents them from shooting a large number of foul shots in a row, a procedure that is of dubious benefit. The coach should also seek to discover ways in which he can exert pressure on the foul shooter during practice sessions. It is generally felt that the key to successful foul shooting in games is the ability to withstand the many pressures that confront the player. This can best be accomplished by practicing foul shooting under pressures that are as similar as possible to the game situation.

Also, participation in drills must be game-like and purposeful (see the section on drills). Selection of drills for use in the practice sessions should be done with the idea of preparing the players for the game situation. It should also be emphasized here that the "crucial moments" found in the basketball game should be given attention in practice, rather than to expect the players to perform well under these conditions during the game without any previous practice exposure to them. Included in such are the last-shot situation, the stall, the desperation press, the crucial jump-ball situation, and the overtime situation. Basketball coaches might take a page from the football coach's notebook in this connection. Football coaches have for years practiced their players in simulated closing moments of the half and the closing moments of the game situations in what is commonly referred to by football coaches as the "two-minute drills."

It is considered to be of great benefit to the basketball coach to have his players "hungry" to participate in the practice session as each afternoon rolls around. When practice sessions are spirited and lively, much more is usually accomplished by the coaches and players than if the players dread to participate in practice because of its length. Also, monotonous and routine practices reduce player learning and subsequent performances. Interest may as a result be dissipated. How effectively the coach organizes the practice sessions is the key factor in helping to determine the attitudes that will prevail among the players at game time.

SAMPLE EARLY SEASON PRACTICE SCHEDULE

3:30 Balls should be on the floor for use by the boys who have come to practice early. The players should concentrate on shooting in pairs from spots on the floor that are likely to be prime shooting areas in the team offense.

4:00 Practice begins—lay up drill is conducted at each end of floor. Then each player passes to shooter, then attempts to mildly harass the shooter.

4:10 One-on-one drill is used for dribbling and defensive practice—players are in four lines—defensive player must keep hands behind back at all times. Change of direction dribble is emphasized.

4:20 Full court three man weave drill is started. Players must make basket at each end before they can stop.

4:30 Full court three on two fast break drills begin.

4:45 Practice begins on one-on-one shooting and defensive drills are conducted at all four baskets.

5:00 Three on three half court offensive drill is organized using a forward, medium high post and a guard. Both ends of floor are used.

5:15 Two on two defensive drill begins with guards. They pick up offensive guards just over the half court line. Centers and forwards work on defensive pivot play at other end of the floor.

5:30 Full court shooting drill is started. Each player must shoot ten jump shots at each end. Every time they cross the half court line, they must take five quick steps to the right, five steps back, five steps to the left and then start for the basket. Three lines are used. Players not involved should shoot free throws at the side basket. They shoot only twice at any one time. A record is kept of the number made and missed.

5:45 Wind sprints—stopping and starting is emphasized.

5:50 Everybody goes to the showers.

Total practice time: One hour and fifty minutes.
Remarks on drills: entered by coach after practice.
Remarks on player performance: entered by coach after practice.

SAMPLE PRACTICE SCHEDULE (MIDDLE OF THE SEASON)

3:30 Early individual instruction and shooting practice is held for boys who can attend practice early. Coach works with Bob on jump shot taken from left hand dribble—works with Walt on short hook shots attempted from either side of the basket—coach checks position of elbow on Gene's jump shot.

4:00 Practice begins—three lane fast break drill is conducted—players concentrate on aggressive rebounding by the three players making the break—two defensive players are used—players should shoot two free throws at side basket before returning to the line.

4:15 Station drills are conducted—forwards break into lane to receive pass and attempt to drive or shoot—centers work on screening out and rebounding with emphasis on initiating fast break with a good outlet pass—guards work on dribbling against heavy defensive pressure.

4:30 Half-court offense is started—particular attention is directed to the weak side play and to movement made by weak side forward—Jerry is used as first substitute at forward—Bill alternates with Bob and Ken at guard.

4:50 Half-court defensive formation is organized. Coach reviews 1-2-2-zone defense for possible use against Tech Friday night—emphasizes the aggressive rush toward the corner and also the weakside wingman rebounding the weakside of the basket—tells the boys where Tech's two good shooters are most likely to play against this zone and emphasizes aggressive coverage of these spots.

5:10 Free throw shooting is begun—two shots at one time taken—all baskets.

5:15 Scrimmage

	Blues	*Whites*
	Ken	Al
	Bob	Gordon
	Walt	Jimmy
	Gene	Shorty
	Russ	Ed

Whites use Tech's switching man-to-man defense and also their zone offense —Blues will play the 1-2-2-zone defense and attempt to fast break at every opportunity.

5:35 Free throws are taken at baskets—the players must make first one to get second attempt.

5:40 Wind sprints are taken.

5:43 All players go to showers.

Total Practice Time: One hour and forty-three minutes.
Remarks on offense and defense: entered by coach after practice.
Remarks on player performance: entered by coach after practice.

SAMPLE PRACTICE SCHEDULE (END OF THE SEASON)

3:30 Only Walt and Bob are to be asked to come to practice early—the coach works with Bob on his change of direction dribble with a drive toward the basket—student manager lobs the ball to Walt in the low post where he should practice short hook shots and jump shots.

4:00 Practice begins—short lay-up practice is undertaken emphasizing *spirit*—the coach emphasizes the fact that there are only two practices left before the first game of the tournament begins.

4:10 The coach reviews offensive pattern of first opponent in tournament—he emphasizes the places in the pattern where shots are most likely to be taken. Individual assignments are made for man to man defense to be used against first tournament opponent.

4:15 Half court defense is practiced—second team runs the opponent's offense. Each member of second team is given a name corresponding to the names of the opponents—the coach emphasizes how and where the players may anticipate the switch on their double screen.

4:40 Half-court offensive formation is practiced—opponents will most likely use a match-up zone defense—the coach emphasizes the continuity of his zone offense—tries to get the forward to look for Walt on the second cut through the lane—makes sure the guards present enough of an offensive threat to prevent the defensive guards from sagging into the lane too far.

5:05 Practice on the stall offense is conducted—the movement of the ball is emphasized.

5:15 Full court practice is held—three-minute drill is begun—score tied and three minutes remaining—free throws are shot in between drills.

5:30 All players go to showers.

Total Practice Time: One hour and thirty minutes.
Remarks on offense and defense: entered by coach after practice.
Remarks on player performance: entered by coach after practice.

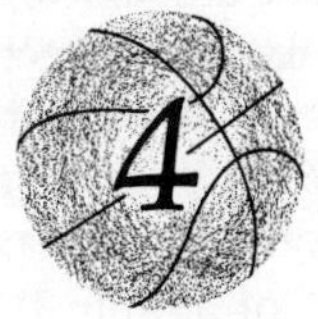

Administration of the Total Basketball Program

Introduction

The basketball coach must be concerned with the total administration of the basketball program if he is continuously to have a successful team. There are many tasks involved in the administration of a successful basketball program. Even though the athletic director may be in charge of most of the administrative phases, the basketball coach must be knowledgeable and concerned about them because they ultimately have an effect on the quality of his program. In some school systems, the athletic director delegates most of the sports administrative responsibilities to the various head coaches and under this administrative arrangement the basketball coach will necessarily be involved in all aspects of the administration of his total program.

It should be stated at the outset that the head coach cannot personally perform all the many administrative tasks that will be given to him. He must learn how to delegate some of them, and then oversee the proper execution of these tasks. There must be a division of responsibility and the proper handling of a particular task will aid the coach in properly fulfilling his administrative responsibilities. It is suggested that each coach prepare a comprehensive and exhaustive list of all the many tasks that he may be confronted with in relation to the successful planning and carrying out of the basketball program. With the use of this list the coach can then attempt to group the tasks into logical categories that will aid him ultimately in delegating some of the tasks to the proper staff members. The coach may discover that several of the tasks are janitorial in nature and he may appoint one person to be responsible for this aspect of the program. He may determine that several of the tasks are directly related to the care and handling of equipment. Thus, he may delegate the responsibility for these tasks to the assistant coach or an equipment manager. The important point to remember is that in this type of administrative procedure the head coach is able (or should be able) to have one person responsible for any given task. When each member of the staff is fully informed as to what is expected of him, he then may perfect his own plans for the fulfillment of these tasks.

At several regularly scheduled times before, during, and after the basketball season the coach may call the entire staff together for meetings at which time certain questions can be answered, problems ironed out, future plans made, and past performances evaluated. If the coach operates in this manner, then he truly should be in command of his total basketball operation. In the remaining portion of this section an attempt is made to acquaint the coach with several important phases of the total basketball program in which he will be administratively engaged. Wherever possible, principles are suggested which could aid the coach in establishing standards to use in improving his basketball system of operation.

Management by Objectives

This text has consistently advocated the use of clear, precise goals and objectives for teaching and coaching basketball. In Chapter 1, under the section, Principles of Motor Learning, as Applied to the Learning of Basketball Skills, clear and precise goals were cited as crucial to developing a proper learning environment for teaching basketball skills and strategies. This concept is even further developed in Chapter 5, where the use of performance objectives is suggested as the best method for teaching basketball in physical education classes. It seems fairly obvious that objectives are necessary for good learning to take place. However, the use of objectives in administering the basketball program may be less evident to the prospective coach.

In the past several decades, business and industry have benefited greatly from what has come to be known as the "management by objectives" approach to administration. Precise goals are set for the organization or business and then performance is measured against these goals. The same basic format can be utilized by the basketball coach to optimize the performance of his total basketball program.

The coach can set personal management goals for himself. For example, he can decide before a season what goals he should achieve in his role as coach. Perhaps he might decide to scout each opponent at least two times, have his team learn at least three basic offensive sets, have a clear plan for each practice, have a clear plan for each game, and provide a post-game feedback session for his team after each game.

The coach can certainly set performance goals for his team. He might set goals in the following areas: (1) turnovers, (2) shooting percentages, (3) rebounds, and (4) points allowed the opponents. Even more sophisticated performance goals can be set. For example, the coach might strive for his team to have an offensive efficiency rating of 1.25. Offensive efficiency is generally defined as the number of points scored divided by the number of times the team brings the ball across the half-court line. Setting team goals like these just mentioned help the players to focus on a group effort, and the feedback about the degree to which they meet the goals provides some measure of group performance and group cohesiveness.

The coach can also set performance goals for each game. For example, the coach might scout a team and decide that his team's defense should force the opponents to shoot the majority of their shots from certain places on the floor. A shot chart can be posted showing the areas where the opponents should shoot from and the percentage of shots that the coach has set as the goal for the game. The shot chart from the actual game can then be rated to see how well the team did in meeting its goal. Again, a major value of this procedure is to help the team focus on important points of strategy and to build a sense of working together toward group goals.

Assistant coaches and managers can also be rated in terms of the degree to which they meet performance objectives which they have set for themselves or have set in conference with the head coach. This helps each member of the organization to have a clear idea of what his role is, what specific tasks he needs to perform to have the program operate well, and also provides a system where performance can be evaluated. Coaches should give serious consideration to using clear, precise objectives in their roles as administrators of the total basketball program.

Scheduling Procedures

The basketball coach is often given the responsibility for scheduling basketball games for his team. However, he must conform to national, state and league regulations that are made concerning scheduling procedures. These regulations will influence and in some instances help determine his ultimate schedule. The following schedule principles are enumerated to help basketball coaches properly plan their basketball schedules within the circumstances mentioned above.

1. It is generally agreed that there should be a limitation on the number of games each team can participate in during the season.

2. Participation in not more than two or three tournaments prior to the play-off tournaments is usually recommended.

3. Usually there should be a restriction on the distance a high school team should travel to play any one game. In areas where this is impossible such as in the desert regions provision should be made for study and conducting classes during the travel time.

4. Home games should not interfere with the regular educational program. That is, school normally should not be dismissed early in order for the game to start before the closing of the school hour.

5. Schedules should be made as far in advance as possible in order to avoid scheduling problems.

6. Most games should be scheduled so that there is equal competition among teams. Educational leaders do not condone uneven contests.

7. An effort should be made to avoid scheduling basketball games at a time when they conflict with other school functions including other team contests.

8. The number of games per week should be limited to not more than two and it may be advisable to conduct the contests only on the weekends.

9. There should be restrictions or elimination of off season and summer practices.

10. The health and welfare of athletes must be considered at all times. Young people should not be asked to play too many games in a short period of time.

11. Confirmation of scheduled games including contractural arrangements should be received well in advance of the date of the game.

Scouting

The act of scouting opponents is an important and necessary aspect of the operational planning that goes into the administration of a competitive basketball program. In some instances the coach may do some of the scouting himself, or he may delegate the performance of this task to an assistant coach, at least part of the time. Some coaches at the university level prefer to have an assistant coach who has as his primary responsibility that of scouting the opposition. An effective job of scouting the opposing teams can aid the coach in properly preparing his offensive and defensive game procedures to be used against the teams on his schedule. It might also provide him with the small, seemingly insignificant pieces of information that may be used in certain situations to bring about the difference between a victory and a defeat.

Two different procedural plans are needed for the performance of the task of scouting. How this is done depends on whether one, two or more scouts are used to view the game. When two scouts are assigned to the task, it is obvious that more information can be accumulated concerning a game than if one is used for this purpose. One scout should keep a chart of the shots taken and made by the players that are being scouted. He should be careful to record accurately the exact positions on the floor where the shots were taken by the players. This same scout might also record the number and kind of floor errors made by the team being scouted. Other information concerning rebounds and assists could be secured by him to aid the head coach in getting an accurate picture of the opposing team's performance. The second scout should be responsible for the recording of all other information needed concerning the team as a whole and specifics about each player. This scout could secure some of this information on the players before the game actually starts. Included in this category should be such items as height, weight, and uniform number of each player. If an adequate form is developed for use in recording this information, the scout can easily add other pertinent data to it concerning each player as the game progresses. This other information might include such items as jumping ability, aggressiveness, dribbling ability, shooting ability, and defensive ability. Some scouts prefer to use a standardized form developed for just such use that allows them merely to write a number signifying the rating given to each of these categories about each player (see scouting report). The coach who is familiar with such a rating system can develop a specific rating list for his use that includes the various abilities he considers important in playing the game of basketball. The use of such a chart would allow the scout to record a maximum amount of information about the opposing players with a minimum amount of effort expended in a minimum amount of time.

This second scout must also be responsible for recording the offensive patterns and plays as well as the type or types of defense that are utilized by the opposing team during the game. This information should be recorded so that an indication is given concerning the time during the game in which the various happenings occurred. For example, a team might change from one defense to another toward the close of the first half and/or near the end of the game. This change in defensive formation would most likely be done to help keep the players from fouling during these crucial moments. The point here is that to secure the information that the team sometimes uses a zone defense (but usually man-to-man defense) is not enough to be of great aid to the coach unless he knows when and why the change was made.

The scout may find that some offensive patterns are easily and quickly

SCOUTING REPORT

Team Scouted: Date:
Place: Opponent:

Personnel

Position	Name	#	Ht.	Wt.	Jump	Dribble	Shoot	Rebound

(Jump, Dribble, Shoot and Rebound are grouped under "Ratings of Players".)

Additional Comments on Personnel:

Diagrams to Use to Record Opponent's Offensive Patterns

Defense

Type of man-to-man defense used:

How aggressive is the man-to-man defense:

Type of zone defense used:

Type of pressing defense used:

Defensive comments and other appropriate statements:

General Information: (typical questions that need to be answered)

Does one player control the ball on offense?

Is the team right handed in its offensive pattern?

What out of bounds plays do they use?

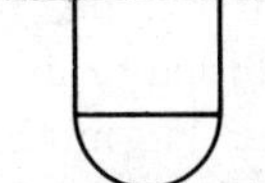

What jump ball plays did they attempt?

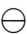

How does the team play against the screening situation?

Can this team be pressed?

Does the team use a stall pattern?

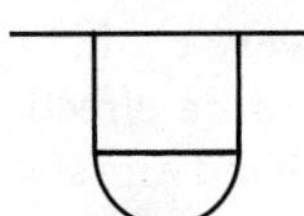

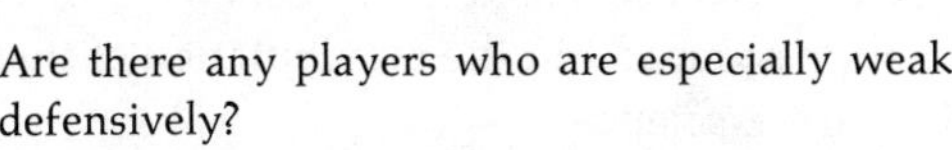

Are there any players who are especially weak defensively?

Are there any players who are hesitant about shooting on offense?

Who is their best free throw shooter?
Worst?

How good of physical condition is the team in?

General Summary:

recorded, while others are so intricate that it may take him a large part of the game time to record them in their entirety.

When only one scout is used, then the shot chart and other statistical information should be omitted from the report. However, specific information about the players and the offensive and defensive information used must be recorded. Yet the single scout should attempt to gain as much information as he can about the game statistics afterwards from radio or newspaper coverage of the game. Also, he should include a box score and a newspaper resumé of the game in his final scouting report if possible.

Regardless of the number of scouts used, it must be emphasized that scouting is as much an art as it is a science since the scout attempts to record accurately the action that takes place during a game. Both aspects are important to the effectiveness of a good scouting report. The art of scouting lies in the ability to sort out and record expertly those pieces of information that are likely to aid the coach the most in his planning for the game. This information also might help the coach in his making of decisions during the actual game. To illustrate, a scout might have noted that one guard has great difficulty in dribbling when he is forced to use his left hand for this purpose. He might also have noticed that one certain player is ineffective in shooting free throws when under pressure. Furthermore, he might have observed that a forward can be intimidated from going to the defensive boards. Also, he might have found out that in the pressure situation a team depends upon only one player to attempt most of the shots taken at the basket. Also, he might have noticed that the pivot player never drives toward the basket, but rather he prefers to shoot fall away, hook, and/or jump shots. Discovery of this type of information makes scouting an art, and thus the scout to be effective must be an experienced basketball observer. On the other hand, the statistical information secured and the manipulation of these raw figures into meaningful data are a science.

Finally, many coaches often want the scout to rely on the use of questions to be assured that he has secured all the necessary information that is needed in the scouting report. A list of such questions and the answers to some of them should be prepared in advance, and checked on periodically during the game to see which ones still remain unanswered. A partial list of representative questions is presented below. It must be stressed that each coach will want to compose his own set of questions, so that he will be sure that he secures the information that he believes is important for use in game planning.

1. Does one player control the ball more than any other player?
2. Is the team right handed in its use of its offensive pattern?
3. What out-of-bounds plays do they use?

4. What jump ball play did they attempt?
5. Is this a fouling team? Which player is most likely to foul?
6. How does the team play against screening situations?
7. Can the team be pressed easily and effectively?
8. Do their players pass the ball against the press or do they dribble it?
9. Do they have a stall pattern that they use?

A summary should be included at the end of the scouting report. It should be prepared sometime after the game, and perhaps not until the next day. It should contain the main impressions that were gained concerning the opposing team and its players. It should include also such general considerations as team aggressiveness, team speed, and team poise.

An actual scouting report made of an opposing team by a top scout at a major university.*

Team Scouted: New York State College
Date: 1/14/74
Opponent: Boston State College
Site: New York State College gymnasium
Scout: John Wright
Halftime score: 40–32 (BC)
Final score: 73–69 (BC)

PERSONNEL

F Larry Jones Jr. 6′4″ 195 lbs. #52

Excellent shot from 12–15′, prefers this shot to the drive
Goes to the offensive board well when a teammate shoots—strong rebounder
Weak defensive player
Plays a wing on offense

F Tom Rice Sr. 6′6″ 205 lbs. #42

He is their workhorse
Works the boards extremely hard
Excellent jumper
Good driver—prefers to go right
Not effective past 12′ distance
Good defensive player
Plays the baseline on offense

*The names of the schools and players have been changed to prevent recognition.

C Ron Cord Jr. 6′8″ 225 lbs. #54

Very quick for his size
Will take the shot from outside but prefers to work inside
Has an effective hook with both left and right hand
Jumps well—hits the boards hard—plays in the middle on offense

G Johnny Stevens Sr. 6′1″ 175 lbs. #24

Left-handed
Good jump shooter—effective from 20–25′
Prefers to go to his left
Very quick
Good ball handler
Penetrates well
He handles the ball most of the time
Plays the point on their offense

G Will Klein Jr.6′ 180 lbs. #32

Only an average shooter
Prefers to pass off
Weak ball handler—can't go left
Good defensive player
Plays a wing on offense

DEFENSIVE BREAKDOWN

They played a man-to-man the entire game. They do a good job of contesting the forwards. They also apply good pressure on the guards, picking up at half court. They will switch G–G or F–F, but never G–F. Basically, they are a good defensive team. They work very hard. Jones, #52 is the weak point of their defense.

MATCH-UP

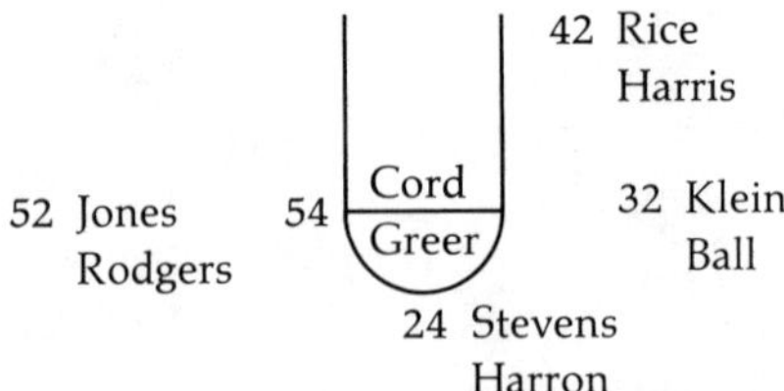

STRATEGY

Defensively, we must:

1. Force Stevens to his right each time he comes down the floor.
2. Make Klein handle the ball on the wing.

3. Keep the ball away from Jones on the other wing.
4. Deny Cord the ball on the high post.

Against their basic patterns:

1. Harris must front Rice at the low post.
2. Hatton must get to the ball side of the screen, then front Stevens.
3. We must deny Cord the ball; Harris must be alert to help from the baseline.
4. Ball and Greer must switch at times.
5. This will be an automatic switch between Ball and Harris. Then Ball will pick up Rice coming off the double pick.

1st Sub Mark Drake 6-1/3″ 190 lbs. #12

Will play either guard or forward
Good shooter from 15′
Drive well
Not a strong rebounder
Will play a wing on offense

OFFENSIVE BREAKDOWN

Boston played a man-to-man defense the entire game
N.Y. ran the following patterns from a 1–3–1 set up

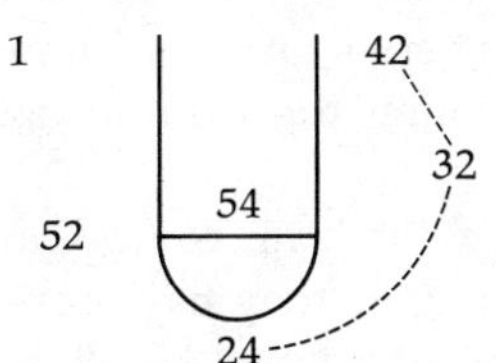

They hit either wing and try to punch the ball directly to the low post

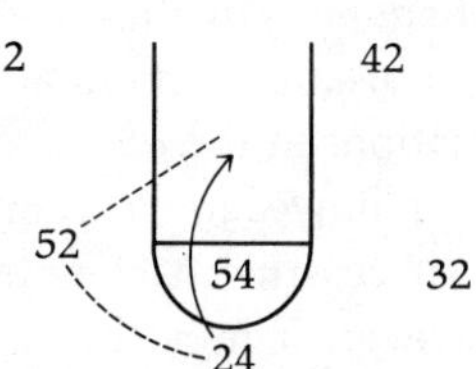

Sometimes 24 will hit the wing and shuffle cut to the basket using 54 for a screen. Will go to either side

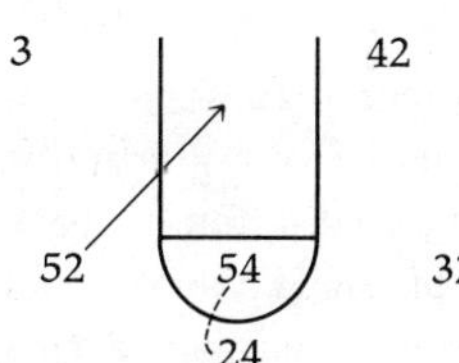

They hit the high post and weakside forward backdoors

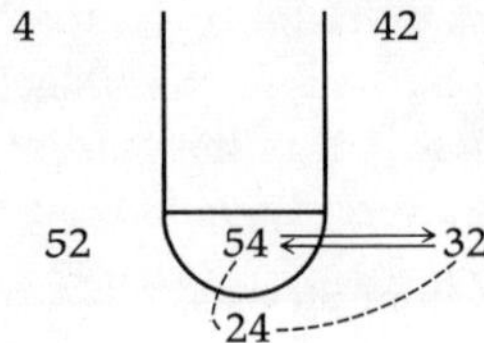

They hit either wing and if he cannot get the ball to baseline, 54 will come to the ball for a basic pick T roll

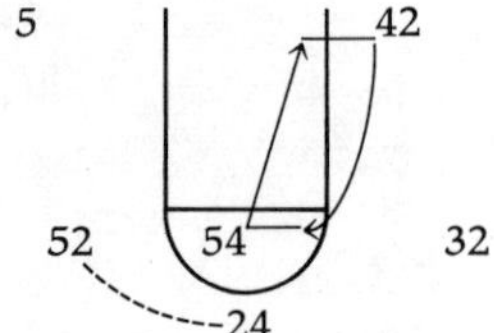

Hit opposite wing 52, 54 + 32 set a double pick for 42 coming to the foul line

Preparing for Tournaments

It has often been a source of wonderment and sometimes consternation to certain coaches as to how a specific coach constantly has his team do well in tournament play. Even when his season's record is very spotty somehow his team manages to go far in tournaments. What accounts for this unusual quality the coach exhibits or his team displays?

Sometimes this coach cares little or not at all how his team comes out in the league standings or pre-tournament play as long as they have confidence and great desire to do well in post-season tournaments. Usually in college conferences and even in some high school leagues only the winners are permitted to participate in the post-season tournaments. In these instances some of the ideas presented here would not be usable. Others are worth considering in connection with the specific situation. In the effort to determine the causes of such fine play some of the steps followed and certain of the ideas and concepts usually fostered by such successful coaches in preparing for tournament play are listed below. However, it must be remembered that there may be many approaches to making proper preparation for tournament play. The coach will have to develop his own ideas after evaluating and experimenting with these and others.

1. Teams often begin to start pointing for tournament play as soon as the season begins. This means the coach brings his squad along gradually. He substitutes often to give game experience to many players, ten at least, and he determines what boys will perform best under stress. This does not mean trying to lose early games, but it does place an emphasis on factors

other than always winning. Development of a defeatist attitude, of course, must be avoided as far as possible. However, a team may be told that they are preparing for the spring tournament(s) during the early part of the season which means both psychological and physical preparation. Thus, almost everything the coach does has a relationship to subsequent tournament competition.

2. The forthcoming schedule must be studied by the coach with the players. He should show them what teams they will play against. He should reveal at least in part what his plans are for the season.

3. The top teams should be scheduled throughout the season if possible to acquaint the players with the good players of these teams. Players learn much more rapidly playing against skilled performers and well drilled teams. They know how well these players can perform and the weaknesses of the top players. It also shows them how much improvement they will have to make before they will be tournament contenders. From a psychological point of view it can be shown to them that if their win and loss record for the season is not too good, it is a result of playing against the very best teams and that such experience will pay off later.

4. Three weeks or a month before tournament play is scheduled to begin, plans are made for the use of detailed strategy and necessary changes are made in playing personnel. Offensive and defensive formations should be stabilized now and practice is begun with the goal of tournament victories kept in mind. Very few last minute changes can be made successfully. Any major tactical changes done at this time make adequate preparation that much more difficult for the players to accomplish.

5. Usually the basic fundamentals are stressed during the entire season. The coach should be constantly stating that under this stressing of the fundamentals program boys who were only mediocre during the season sometimes are able to become top performers by tournament time.

6. The squad usually adopts strict but feasible training rules and those who do not care to abide by them are dropped from the squad. What these rules are will vary from locality to locality and from coach to coach. However, they usually involve some sacrifice on the part of the players. Some of these rules involve: establishing a definite time to eat; understanding and adhering to proper eating and drinking habits; having regular hours of sleep; restricting dating procedures; adhering to agreed upon procedures to follow for the night before a game, for after school time and before game night; agreeing as to the time to eat the before-game meal; deciding on the arrival time for the game and what will be acceptible as an excuse; determining as to the proper personal conduct desired relative to smoking and drinking, etc. These are among the items the squad may establish as rules and regulations that are to be followed by all members.

7. Practice and play if possible have been conducted on the same court or one similar to the one where the tournament is to be scheduled. At least, the team should try to play one or more games during the season on the tournament court if it is possible.

8. Players must be familiar with many styles and types of offenses and defenses. This needed experience may be gained through playing teams from various sections of the region. The opposing teams using more than one style of defense and offense help acquaint them with the advantages and disadvantages of the use of different styles. The players in turn should be better equipped to cope with the many styles of play, regardless of what style(s) of play a team uses. During the regular season, some time in pre-tournament practice should be spent in getting acquainted with the most common styles likely to be used by other teams in the tournament.

9. Experience gained with the officiating procedures used in many sections aids in preparation. If the names of the officials for the tournament are known beforehand and the team is definitely unfamiliar and not accustomed to their style(s), it would be wise to have some local official imitate them by officiating a practice session if it can be arranged.

10. Most coaches like to arrange one or two overnight trips during the season to take the edge off of this exciting experience and to condition the players for this type of experience.

11. During the season periodic review is made concerning how the teams throughout the county, region, and state are faring—who the top teams are and what seems to be their style of play, who does their scoring, etc., if such information can be obtained. A visit(s) by the squad to observe top play by good teams, both high school and college, should be encouraged.

12. An occasional scrimmage with the town team, or college "B" team (a college team could practice against an A.A.U. team) can be helpful if such a team is not too superior or too much rough play does not ensue and if the rules governing play permit this type of arrangement to take place.

13. The last week before the tournament, practice should be somewhat shorter than usual, but conducted at a fast tempo. Mental attitude now is more important than last minute work on skills.

14. As soon as it becomes known who the first opponent will be in the tournament, practice on procedures designed for use against this team should be started. Using the last one or two practices for the purpose of preparing the home team for its first opponent is usually too late. Mental and physical preparation should have been started earlier before the attention of the players has been distracted by the thoughts of the trip.

15. Arrangement should be made to have the players stay at home as long as possible before going to the tournament. If the distance to the tournament is not too long, it is believed it would be better to drive back

and forth each day until the team is eliminated. However, a trip that lasts more than three hours in a car is too long to make each day.

16. Tournament plans and a time schedule to be followed are made out well in advance for use during the actual tournament competition. Certain suggestions are made here which have been found by several top coaches to be profitable. They are as follows:

a. The players should practice on some fundamentals briefly before each game.

b. The coach must be careful not to make great changes in the established offensive and defensive patterns.

c. The team should prepare for and play each game as it comes up. The players should not look ahead to the playing of some team one or two games hence.

d. The players should be kept occupied between games; not permitted to run around or to sleep continuously. Plenty of rest and sleep should be gotten at about the same time as at home.

e. Players should be allowed enough money in order to secure the proper amount of food, but eating between meals should be restricted. A place that serves good meals should be selected in advance.

f. The amount of time spent in watching the other games should be curtailed. Two games in a morning would usually be enough for the day if the team is playing a game at night.

g. The players should eat, sleep, and live in as nearly like home conditions as possible.

h. The amount of visiting home fans can do with the players should be limited. Housing the boys in a part of the hotel (if not at home) where street and hotel traffic is the least is recommended.

i. A study should be conducted on how to arrange the sleeping mates so that the least amount of talking in bed results. Some coaches prefer to have close friends room together, others want room-mates to be players who are not close friends.

j. The coach must be wary of carrying out suggestions about team play given him by vocal but well meaning town folks. The coach is hired to make decisions regarding the planned maneuvers and selection of playing personnel. Fathers sometimes upset their playing sons by their unintentional interference. The coach should try to avoid the occurrence of such parental obstruction. Preventing a lot of visiting with the players by any outsiders helps reduce the possibility of this happening.

k. The team should practice the night before the tournament begins at the site if at all possible.

The establishment of a visiting period may satisfy parents, town folks and players. However, each coach must decide in advance the relative importance of some of these items and make his plans accordingly. Many coaches establish a procedure that is a happy medium between having their team do well during the season and play well in the post-season tournaments. Under this policy the planning should involve winning the big games during the season when it counts the most, yet also be pointing the team for tournament play. Some of the ideas proposed in this section could be used in planning for just such an approach.

Pre-Game Check List

In most situations regardless of who is delegated the responsibility for or undertakes to perform the various pre-game duties, the head basketball coach in the final analysis is the responsible person. This applies to a goal that needs a new net; a slick place found on the floor. Maybe the student manager or the janitor had been assigned the duty to check on these things. However, the game is ready to start and for some reason no one did check and the game is delayed while an embarrassed coach hurriedly performs a task that should have been done earlier.

It is for the purpose of helping to avoid such happenings as mentioned above that a sample pre-game check list has been prepared. It is recognized that each situation is so different that only a suggestive check list can be presented here. Yet it is believed that many of the items listed are common to most situations. Such a mimeographed check list should be available for use for each game. Those persons who have been assigned certain duties and responsibilities should make a check by those items for which they have accepted responsibility so that it is evident that they have completed their assignments.

It is not enough that items are glanced at on the check list. Someone must have personally counted the quantity or made the repair and declared that everything is in order for the game.

It is believed that an extensive check list is needed so that no important item will be overlooked. However, the check list must be one that can be quickly read and checked off rapidly.

Certain of the items, such as securing a physician to be present at the game, must be done at least several days in advance. Some may even be done the week before the contest, while others may be done an hour before the game is scheduled to start.

The following check list, though not at all inclusive, contains a large number of items thought to be important to the proper conduct of the basketball game.

SUGGESTED PRE-GAME BASKETBALL CHECK LIST

____

(Date)

I. *Facilities, Equipment and Supplies*

Inflation of game balls to proper pressure is done.

The floor was cleaned the afternoon of the game.

Blackboard and chalk are placed in the visitors' quarters.

The visitors' quarters are clean and warm.

The officials' quarters are clean and warm.

The visitors' showers are clean and equipped with soap and towels.

The officials' showers are clean and equipped with soap and towels.

The temperature at court level is proper.

The visitors' colors do not conflict with the home team's. (An extra set of jerseys may need to be available.)

Warm water for after game showers for the home players, officials, and visitors will be available.

Ventilation in the gymnasium is adequate.

Game uniforms are laid out by number and name before the players arrive for the contest.

The scoreboard is functioning properly.

The scorebook is ready for use.

The clock is running properly.

All lights will turn on.

Whistles and extra shirts are available for officials.

A stop watch is available in case the official clock fails.

The scorer's table is in the proper place in the gymnasium.

The timer's horn is on the table (or the timer's gun is on the table and will work).

The first aid kit is ready for use.

All unnecessary apparatus is off the playing floor.

Good nets are on the goals.

The goals and boards are firm, nothing is broken.

The loud speaker system is hooked up and working.

The officials are informed of the local ground rules concerning the playing court.

II. *Management of Personnel*

All managers have indicated that they will be present: Senior, "B" squad, Freshman, etc.

Confirmation from officials as to date and time of game has been received.

The visiting team has been notified of the starting time.

The janitor has been told to admit managers and players early.

Statisticians are available.

The visiting team has been notified as to the names of the officials for the game.

Training room helpers have been assigned and told when to report, *i.e.* towel man, water boy, etc.

Provisions have been made for paying the officials.

An alternate official is available.

Timers have been assigned.

The scorer has been assigned.

Ticket takers have been assigned (may be done by vice-principal).

Ticket sellers are available.

Tickets are on hand.

Change money is available.

Complimentary tickets have been designated.

The program has been printed and delivered.

The physician has been contacted and has accepted.

Ushers are assigned.

III. *Players*

They have been told when to report.

Names of those suiting up for the game have been posted.

The time for eating has been stated.

Provisions have been made for early taping and the specific players notified.

Energy helpers (such as sugar, oranges) are available.

IV. *Trip out of Town*

Transportation has been arranged in advance (bus and driver, plane, private car).

The time of departure is posted.

The names of the players making the trip are posted.

Designation of managers to make the trip has been done.

Parental consent or release has been secured.

Arrangement has been made for issuance and transportation of game equipment.

Spare wearing apparel is packed.

Practice balls are packed.

Meal arrangements are provided for if necessary.

Parents are notified of the approximated time of return.

Opponent's gymnasium floor has been checked.

Timer and scorer are arranged for the game.

First aid equipment is available.

Purchase and Care of Equipment

The purchase and care of equipment are an important item in the proper administration of the basketball program. In some situations the basketball coach has all the responsibility in this connection. In others his suggestions and recommendations constitute all he may do. However, concerning equipment, regardless of who has the responsibility, the purshase and proper care of basketball equipment may materially affect the way the team(s) performs. Certainly a shoddily dressed team practicing with a ball that does not bounce correctly is having to work under a handicap.

PURCHASE

There are many general principles that might be established to aid in purchasing basketball equipment. Two, however, may be stated here as being important:

1. Improvement of service to the students is the goal. This would mean that equipment was supplied to all students (at least all team players) if possible. Equipment would be of the best quality for these students.

2. The most economical use of available funds is made. Purchase of certain grade balls (although they may be official) may be more economical in the long run than the purchase of another grade. Uniforms of a more or a less expensive type may be purchased and may prove to be more economical over a five- or ten-year period than another.

The above general principles form the foundation upon which specific guiding principles of buying may be established. Some of these guiding principles are listed below:

1. Equipment purchases should conform to specifications. If the establishment of specifications has come about after careful planning, then acceptance of equipment below or even above what is desired is usually not a good business procedure.

2. Equipment to be purchased should be of a high quality. It almost always pays to purchase top quality equipment if cost of operation is determined over a five- or ten-year period. High quality type of goods usually lasts longer than cheaper equipment when a cost ratio is considered.

3. The price paid for basketball equipment usually should be consistent with market conditions and prices. An article that appears to be equal to other standard brands but is way below the going market price should be scrutinized closely before being bought. The "good buy" should be carefully examined before being purchased.

4. The purchase of large quantities of equipment is usually recommended. The larger the quantity, the cheaper an individual item will be. Planned purchasing on an annual or biennial basis often permits quantity buying. However, styles of equipment become outmoded and care should be exercised that equipment will not have to be discarded before it is used for a sufficient length of time. Some equipment, such as rubber, deteriorates on the shelf and for this reason large quantities should not be bought and stored for future use.

5. A purchase order should be submitted early before the market is flooded. Submission of a purchase order in late August or September may be too late for safe delivery. Usually the purchase orders should be prepared early in the spring for delivery in September. However, sometimes prices change and it may be profitable to wait until summer to submit purchase orders. Discussion of this point with representatives from reputable firms may help in arriving at the right decision.

6. The securing of legitimate discounts should be the goal of the purchaser. Payment of bills made before a certain date usually merits a discount with some companies. This is a saving worth consideration. On the other hand, acceptance by the purchaser of special discounts, concessions and gifts from the seller obligates not only the purchaser, but the school he represents and should be avoided.

7. Reputable firms and full time salesmen should usually be patronized. Established companies usually make good on faulty equipment, but unstable firms cannot afford to refund money or replace inferior equipment. New salesmen should be carefully evaluated because sometimes they are not completely familiar with their companies' policies and even their equipment. It is recommended that a clear understanding on contractual arrangements be made with the home office before orders are submitted.

8. Usually one company has a special type of equipment they feature (or manufacture). It is possible for their representative to know more about this one item than salesmen from other companies. It is usually good business to purchase these featured articles from the known manufacturer. However, it is also good business to buy from more than one firm, usually several of the best firms. This competition invites good service and helps keep the salesmen and firms on the lookout for new ideas. In addition, the school is not obligated to any firm, and companies know they must furnish good equipment in order to keep the school's business.

9. The habit of buying under salesmanship pressure usually should be avoided. Equipment should be purchased after the buyer has seen the latest innovations from several companies. Time should be given over to reflection and evaluation before final purchase orders are submitted. Especially is this true when major items are purchased.

10. An accurate inventory of all equipment should be made prior to the placing of any orders. Making use of an inaccurate inventory may result in needless buying.

11. In order to avoid mistakes and misunderstandings between the purchaser, the school administration and the seller, accurate records of all negotiations must be kept. This usually means that each order is made out in triplicate so that all parties have a copy.

12. Defective goods and those not meeting specifications should be

returned immediately. It sometimes happens that a part of a shipment is defective or short in numbers, but the mistake is not discovered until after part of the equipment has been used. A thorough check and count should be made immediately of all equipment received in a given shipment. Reputable firms will correct any errors that their company has made if the error is reported soon enough.

13. Samples of equipment in correct styles should be tried out by at least some member of the team that will wear them before an order is placed. Players are sometimes very dissatisfied with certain styles and types and this annoying factor could have been eliminated if proper planning had taken place.

CARE

Several hundred dollars can be saved each year by a school district or college if proper care and repair of equipment are made. Certain rules and regulations need to be established so a plan for proper care can be formulated. Some of these rules and regulations are:

1. One person needs to be in charge as stock clerk of all physical education and athletic equipment. This is necessary if accurate records are to be kept. A sample form for keeping such records is shown here. If it is not possible to have a full time clerk or custodian, one person still must be responsible for the keeping of all records.
2. It may be necessary (if a school has a limited budget) to have a custodian present only when equipment is issued to the team.
3. A constant up-to-date inventory of equipment should be made in order to know if any equipment has been stolen and how much has been discarded.
4. A stock room where equipment can be stored in a neat arrangement is needed.
5. If possible, let the custodian or clerk be the only one who has access to the stock room. Coaches, instructors, players, managers only confuse the record keeper if permitted entrance.
6. Some method should be established so that all equipment is returned when the season or year is up. Marking equipment such as "T" shirts with "Stolen from RUHS" sometimes is effective in keeping student from wearing them illegally. A tradition can be established that the equipment is legitimate property of the school and as such must be returned. However, the equipment marked in certain ways can also aid in its becoming a school status symbol, and thus encourage its theft.
7. Any equipment taken from the equipment room must be signed for by the proper people. A procedure is needed to enforce its return or to secure

INVENTORY RECORD OF EQUIPMENT

Date of Inventory: Sport:

Person in charge of inventory: Head coach:

Item of Equipment	Number of items accounted for at last inventory	Number of items purchased since last inventory	Total number of items now available	Number of items in good condition	Number of items in fair condition	Number of unusable items	Number of items needed for next season

proper payment for the loss. Grades, diplomas, and sweaters should be held up until proper accounting is made of all checked out equipment.

Public Relations

One of the responsibilities of the coach is the development of proper public relations. In the most literal sense, the coach "relates" to the public in many ways. While a coach does not necessarily have to be a promoter, to refuse to recognize the fact that public relations is an important aspect of his coaching duties is both incorrect and often disastrous. Indeed, if the coach is aware of the many ways in which he relates to the public, he can do his school and his profession a real service by approaching the public in an honest, enthusiastic, and a dignified manner that will help enhance the educational image of his profession and his school.

The coach should be aware of several general aspects of public relations that are essential to his future success. For example, the coach should always be honest in his reports to the public, but he should not be forced to comment on matters that he believes should not be discussed publicly. The coach should not give the news media representatives what they want if this means hedging on the truth or sensationalizing on something that is obviously not sensational. Also, the coach should never discuss personal matters concerning his players before an audience. Further, the coach should never run down or degrade the opposing team, coach, or its players. This would be a display of both bad manners and poor strategy. Such action gives the opponents a psychological gimmick that might help arouse them to perform above their ability. The coach should also be loyal to his conference and to his sport. Thus, the coach should give due recognition to those who aid in the organization and administration of the total basketball program at his school. It is particularly important that he recognize publicly the contributions of his assistant coaches. The coach should always be courteous to the visiting teams when they come to his school to play against his team. This might include meeting the team and the coaches when they arrive and assigning an assistant manager or a letter winner to act as an official host for the visiting team while they are on his campus.

Whether the coach likes it or not, his behavior during the game is also a matter of public concern. Perhaps it is the most important part of his public relations function. His conduct on the bench and in handling his players is closely observed, especially now that so many of the games are shown on television. For example, to degrade a boy publicly for a mistake he made or for his poor performance on the court is inexcusable. When a boy needs to be "dressed down," he should at least enjoy the right to have this occur in the privacy of the locker room, and preferably in the coach's office. The coach's behavior toward the officials is also a matter of public record. The coach must realize that the players and the fans will take their cues from him in regards to formulating their behavior toward the officials. Generally speaking, the coach who treats his players with respect will be creating the right image. The degree of friendliness a coach displays toward his players is another matter, and is one that should be decided upon by the individual coach in accordance with his philosophy of coaching.

Other aspects of the public relations portion of the coach's job are more formal and business-like. The coach should institute a program involving continuous press releases. It is helpful if the coach can delegate this responsibility to someone connected with the journalism or sports publicity department in his school. The college coach usually will have access to members of the college news bureau to do this task for him and he should use them to great advantage in this respect. In larger colleges and universities an athletic publicity director handles most of these chores.

A brochure should be sent out to all opponents and news media representatives before the opening of the season. This brochure should have a colorful design and should contain a great deal of information about the team, its personnel, and the school. A special program should also be prepared for use at each home game. These types of programs range all the way from mimeographed line-up sheets to colorful and attractive booklets in which the reader is brought up-to-date information about the game and the progress of the team. Often local advertisers are happy to buy space in this type of program, and in turn this income can help defray the expenses of printing it in a professional manner. The proper use of a good program can be a source of enjoyment to the fans and a vital means of gaining good public relations for the school.

Finally, the coach must recognize that he has a prominent position in the community. He will be called upon to participate in many community affairs and to speak at many community gatherings and club meetings. In this way the coach can develop proper public relations by being present at these activities. However, the coach must decide where he is to draw the line on the amount of participation he does in community affairs. He has an obligation to perform his assigned duties as a teacher at his school. Also, most likely he has family obligations that should be met. Thus, he must constantly strive to maintain a balanced approach between home life and participation in these activities. Otherwise he will be unable to perform any of his duties and responsibilities effectively.

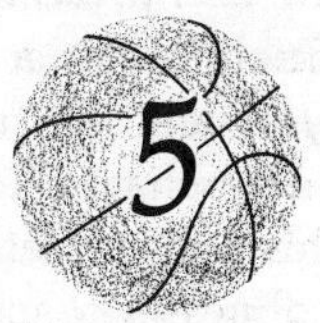

The Basketball Class in Physical Education

Teaching or Coaching

A teacher and a coach of basketball have much the same position in the school in a sense, with each having somewhat the same purposes in mind. There are no real main differences in how each goes about accomplishing the established objectives except in degree unless there are outside influences. From an educational viewpoint every student, whether out for the varsity basketball team or enrolled in a physical education class, should receive the best possible basketball instruction in keeping with his interests and capabilities.

A basketball coach who devotes all of his time and energy to developing varsity players and little toward teaching basketball to the members of his physical education classes is guilty of dereliction of duty. He should get another job or certainly refrain from teaching basketball to students in the physical education classes.

Many potential basketball players are enrolled in the physical education classes. Purely from a selfish viewpoint, it would be a good investment for the basketball coach to give the best instruction possible to all students in the class. He may have need of some of these potential players later on. Also, those who do not make the team may become taxpayers and boosters after graduation. Their support of the school athletic program is needed.

However, there are certain small differences that often exist in the teaching as contrasted with the coaching environment due to the length of the training period, the students' objectives, and the present and future utilization of the skills acquired by the students. Thus, the student out for a varsity team often has a different perspective toward playing basketball than does the regular physical education student.

The following table lists some of the differences that may exist in presenting the basketball program to the student in the physical education class in comparison with doing so to the varsity team candidate:

The only differences are in emphasis and intensity—like a band director—all week practice everyone—game time recital, etc., only play the best.

Coaching a Team	*Teaching a Physical Education Class*
a. Students will have great enthusiasm if properly motivated.	*a.* All students will not have all the enthusiasm that is desired.
b. The student objective is to make the team so he will sacrifice much time and effort to do so.	*b.* Student objectives are different. He is taking a course so he will have to be "sold."
c. If the drills are meaningful, they can be used often with these students.	*c.* Drills should be used, but for only a short time each session.
d. As their skills and performances improve, students want more detailed information on how to perform better.	*d.* Usually the student wants less detail. He may sometimes resist the detailed presentation until he is shown why.
e. Students are more interested in improving than in always playing and readily respond in most instances to any devices used to help them improve.	*e.* Students are often more interested in playing, need something to motivate them to improve, *e.g.*, progressive charts, self-evaluation forms, etc.
f. Students are easy to control and organize because of the fewer numbers and greater interest.	*f.* The class has to be well organized or confusion exists.
g. Students are capable of more self-direction.	*g.* Seniors in high school and college students should be given the opportunity for self-direction. Usually the teacher must direct entire group in participation in drills when dealing with younger or beginning groups.
h. Coaches have usually been motivated to do the best possible instructional job and as a consequence, both pupils and teacher usually work at capacity.	*h.* The philosophy of teaching during the class period is that it is a period of instruction, not necessarily play. Yet through play instruction has meaning. It may be that in the past, instruction has not been meaningful enough so that the student would rather just play the game and learn through trial and error rather than listen to the instructor on how to improve his performance.

Choice of Teaching Methodology

Many suggestions about coaching in this book have been developed directly from theory and research findings from the field of psychology of learning. Indeed, an entire section (see Chapter 1) has been devoted to principles of learning as they apply to coaching basketball. Also, a section (see Chapter 2) has been devoted to principles for the development and selection of drills. Obviously, a teacher/coach could decide to teach basketball in a physical education class much in the same way he coaches; *i.e.* his teaching method and coaching method would be quite similar. If a teacher/coach feels that this is the best method to use, then it is believed there is ample information in this text to provide a sound methodological basis for teaching basketball in physical education classes.

However, as has been already pointed out, the factors that motivate the teacher/coach may differentially affect his performance in teaching as opposed to his performance in coaching. For example, how often does it occur that a basketball coach would allow an assistant to take over a varsity practice so that he could attend a faculty meeting? On the other hand, would the same person be more likely to assign his teaching responsibilities to another teacher for the same purpose? Without wanting to belabor the point, it is simply unrealistic to expect that a teacher/coach will have equal motivation in physical education as contrasted with athletics. This is not to suggest that this is inappropriate. It is only to recognize the realities of the teaching and coaching situation.

Because of the realities of the teaching situation, it may be necessary for a teacher/coach to utilize different methods in the physical education class than in coaching. It is obvious that student interests and motivation will be different in physical education. It is just as obvious that the coach's interests and motivations are different. Because of these factors it is felt that the use of a more highly structured approach to the teaching of basketball might prove beneficial to the teacher/coach. By structuring the physical education class, the teacher/coach can better insure that learning will occur and also that he will have acquitted his responsibilities adequately as a teacher.

Structuring the physical education class does not mean the creation of a rigid learning environment. Rather, it refers to careful planning for the establishment of learning objectives. It is suggested that the teacher/coach consider seriously the widespread utilization of behavioral objectives as an aid to planning and structuring basketball classes in physical education.

Behavioral Objectives for Basketball

A behavioral objective is simply a clear statement of what the student is to learn. The purpose of a performance objective is to communicate to the learner the nature of the learning task, the situation in which the task is to be performed, how the task will be evaluated, and the standard for completion of the task. Aims and goals for the class may be stated in general terms, but performance objectives must refer specifically to what the student is expected to learn.

In teaching basketball, it is standard procedure to list as an objective, for example, the learning of the execution of the chest pass. Simply stating that the chest pass should be learned is not sufficient. In order to develop an acceptable performance objective for this skill, the teacher/coach needs to specify the conditions under which the chest pass is to be made and the standard by which the skill will be judged. To whom does the student make the pass? How far away is the receiver? What if the receiver has to move to catch the ball? How high can the pass go? How many successful passes must be completed to pass successfully a task? Good performance objectives would answer each of these questions. Consider the following performance objective for the chest pass.

Standing 15 feet from a wall, the student will make 9 of 10 chest passes that hit within a 3-foot square target on the wall and go no higher than 6 feet.

This performance objective tells the student exactly what must be done. It also provides a method by which the student can judge his own performance and his progress towards the completion of the task. The performance objective emphasizes accuracy and also a good firm pass. The accuracy is insured by having to hit within a target area. The crispness of the pass is insured by not allowing any pass to go higher than 6 feet.

All of the basic skills of basketball can be easily stated in performance objectives. This is true for passing, dribbling, shooting, rebounding, and more general skills such as quick lateral movement. Furthermore, a progression of skill can be established within each skill area. Dribbling means many things. Performance objectives might be written that emphasize control, speed, speed plus control, dribbling without watching the ball, dribbling with the non-preferred hand, changing direction with the dribble, dribbling behind the back, dribbling against moderate pressure, and dribbling against strong pressure. Each of these tasks can be graded in difficulty simply by changing the standard by which the performance is judged or by changing the situation in which the skill is performed. For example, it would be easy to write a progression of three objectives which emphasized speed in dribbling simply by lowering a time criterion for judging the completion of the tasks. In this way, a basic curriculum of basketball skills could be developed and utilized throughout the physical education program. A few sample objectives are stated below.

Sample Performance Objectives for Basketball

Receiving a pass from a teammate, the student will perform a reverse pivot and make a bounce pass to a second teammate so that the second teammate can receive the pass without having to break a running stride.

Starting from the left wing, the student will dribble to the edge of the lane and shoot a jump shot. Making three of five will constitute passing this task.

The student will dribble the length of the court, changing hands at least three times, and complete the dribble within 10 seconds without incurring a walking or double dribble violation.

The student will dribble the length of the court without committing a violation and without watching the ball.

The student will record a minimum of 60% of 20 free throws per day for three consecutive classes.

Given a diagram of a zone defense, the student will place offensive players in position to combat that defense.

Given a written description of a violation situation, the student will correctly label the violation and describe the penalty imposed.

The student will maintain defensive position against an opponent's dribble for half the court without using his arms.

These examples show the benefit of using performance objectives. The task is stated clearly. The teacher will not have to act as a traffic director during class. Students will understand what they have to do, where they are to do it, and when they have done it well. The standard of performance is clearly stated. This allows the student to utilize the feedback intrinsic in the task to evaluate his own performance. It also allows the student to chart his own progress along the progression of tasks that constitute the skills portion of the class. These are substantial benefits for the student. There is also a substantial benefit for the teacher. He will be sure that some real skill is being developed in his class, and he will have no qualms about having acquitted himself in a thoroughly professional manner.

Behavioral objectives can be utilized in physical education classes for boys or girls. They also would prove very helpful in age-group basketball programs, where there are unusually large numbers of youngsters who need a structured program in order to acquire skills quickly. Naturally, the objectives would be written quite differently for these different situations. The basic skills would remain the same throughout all situations, but the conditions under which the skills are to be performed and the standards for evaluating the skills would be changed so as to be consistent with the developmental level of the students.

Motivation in Teaching Basketball in Physical Education

Normally, a majority of students will be highly motivated in physical education classes in which basketball is the activity. Normal motivation can be enhanced through the use of behavioral objectives. Completing a performance task is rewarding to most youngsters. Likewise, progress towards the completion of a series of tasks is also rewarding, especially if the teacher keeps a progress chart in the gymnasium or locker room so the evidence of progress is public. However, there may be times when special motivational techniques are needed to keep students working hard and to allow for proper functioning of the class as a whole. At the high school level, the grading system might provide some motivation. If performance objectives are used, then the grading system can be quite easily tied to the completion of a specified set of objectives. The basketball teacher can specify "C" level objectives, "B" level objectives, and "A" level objectives. The very same system could be used in age-group basketball programs but instead of grades, the basketball teacher could use designations such as "beginner," "advanced," and "All-star." Age-group swimming programs have made effective use of these motivational techniques for many years and they have proven to be quite successful.

An example of the use of performance objectives tied to a motivational system is offered below. This system of motivation is referred to as "contingency management" and has been shown to be quite effective in many different educational systems. In the illustration below, the tasks are specified in "areas" and the performance criteria are separated into "standard" and "quality" levels.

Example of Contingency Management Plan for Basketball*

	Standard Performance	Quality Performance
AREA 1 Rules Test	Pass with 70%	Pass with 80%
AREA 2 Participation	7 days practice, 1 of which is full court	11 days practice 1 of which is full court

*McDonald, L. J., "An elective curriculum," *Journal of Health, Physical Education and Recreation*, 29, September, 1971.

AREA 3 Shooting		
1. Short shots, any technique	6 baskets in 30 sec.	10 baskets in 30 sec.
2. Free throws, any technique	1 out of 4	2 out of 4
AREA 4 Passing		
1. Chest pass to target (1 block in wall, chest high, 10′ from wall	5 accurate passes in 10 seconds	8 accurate passes in 10 seconds
2. Two-hand overhead throw to wall and catch from 5′ restraining line (no batting)	8 passes in 10 seconds	12 passes in 10 seconds
AREA 5 Dribbling		
Dribble alternately around 4 markers placed 8′ apart and start to first marker is 5′ start to fourth marker is 45′	14.0 seconds	12.1 seconds
AREA 6 Playing ability	Instructor rated	
AREA 7 Officiating		
1. Pass rules test with 90%		
2. Officiate tests		
3. Officiate 4 days, 1 of which is an official game		
4. Instructor's recommendation		

Grades are not the only motivators, however, and they may not be the best. Most boys and girls enjoy playing basketball. They enjoy playing games. They enjoy playing 1 against 1 or 2 against 2. They enjoy doing trick shots and fancy dribbling. A basketball teacher can use these enjoyable activities as motivators. For example, suppose that a teacher has set up a series of drills to use in perfecting skills or a series of performance objectives accomplished by his students. The teacher would like the students to learn these skills as quickly and as efficiently as possible. To do this, he needs to motivate the students to put forth their highest effort. This can be done quite simply by arranging a favorite activity as a reward for completing a specified set of performance objectives. For example, a player can earn 30 minutes of game playing time after successfully completing 10 performance objectives. Or, a player can practice trick shots or play 1 against 1 after completing several more objectives. An easy way to manage the class in this manner is simply to award "free time" as a reward for completing certain objectives. The teacher can then specify 3 or 4 activities that the students can participate in during free time. If these activities are the favorite activities of the students, they will be strongly motivated to learn the skills in order to earn the free time.

Personal conduct is also a matter of importance for basketball teachers. Establishment of proper personal conduct rules to be followed by students is necessary. In order for the class to function smoothly, there are certain rules that must be followed. These rules will vary with the school, age of the students, and even with individual instructors. However, the principle of establishing some rules is a general procedure that should be followed. This is really a problem in motivation. Students know how to behave well. They know how to listen, how to treat equipment properly, how to cooperate and treat other students decently. However, it is just as obvious that they also know how to behave badly. They push and shove in line rather than watching their classmates perform. They mistreat equipment that is becoming more and more expensive to replace. The problem is to make sure that they are motivated enough to behave well rather than to behave poorly. This obviously can be done simply by threatening or coercing the students. However, this text has consistently suggested that positive motivational techniques are superior.

The first step is then to establish rules. Students need to know exactly what is allowed and exactly what is not allowed in the gymnasium and locker room. These rules could even be stated in a manner similar to the performance objectives. The type of motivation used to establish use of the rules depends a great deal on the type of student. If the students are fairly normal in terms of their behavior, then the teacher can usually establish a high degree of good behavior simply by occasionally complimenting individuals or the class when they behave properly. That seems like a simple thing for a teacher to do, but all research findings indicate that it does not occur often enough. When a student has behaved well, an occasional pat on the back or a kind word will usually be sufficient to keep that student behaving well for a long time.

If a poorly behaved class is encountered, good behavior can usually be included in the performance objectives for the class and then tied to the particular reward system. In other words, in order to earn the right to participate in favorite activities the students need not only to learn the skills, but also to behave appropriately. Things such as punctuality, attentiveness to the instructor, and proper care of equipment can easily be written into a contingency management plan.

Principles of Class Organization

It is believed that general adherence to the methods outlined in this chapter and throughout the book would produce a highly satisfactory environment for learning basketball skills in physical education classes and age-group competition. The potential for learning increases with the use of specific objectives, clear rules for behavior, and attention to the motivation of the class. It can also be stated that this kind of sound positive teaching method produces an atmosphere that is the most fun for both the student and the teacher. Several other points are worthy of emphasis. They can aid the teacher in making best use of the methods suggested here.

1. All the members of the class should be kept active even during scrimmages. This is true even when there are too many students to permit them all to be on the floor at the same time. If the class is unusually large to adhere to this principle, this will take a lot of improvising and careful previous planning on the part of the instructor.

Group drills instead of individual drills may be used. Small areas of the court(s) could constitute team boundaries. Basketball and proper falling procedures may be participated in at the same time. Team and group passing may be conducted on the areas adjacent to the court(s). Constant rotation of students in skill practice units may be necessary to keep interest.

2. Proper orientation is given to all student leaders. If it is possible to have a short 5-minute meeting after school, before class, at noon, before school, etc., with the student leaders to discuss plans, their attitude toward their responsibility will often be very favorable. Their attitude in turn will help to get the basketball unit off to a good start. Since most students enjoy participating in basketball, the instructor will usually have to spend less time in orienting the class than in most other sports classes. Explanation can come from the student leaders in casual informal association with the class members rather than in formal sessions conducted by the instructor.

3. Punctuality. The instructor should expect punctuality from the students. A class that is organized so that everyone knows when it begins and ends calls for prompt movement of the students from one class to another. An instructor who expects punctuality on the student's part, but continuously disregards it as it applies to him personally, is not being realistic. Promptness begets promptness.

4. Equating and Equalizing Competition. Students must have some experience in participating against players better than they are skillwise. However, most boys in the physical education class would become discouraged and lose interest in playing if the caliber of play of the players that they participate against is superior to their ability all the time. They need to feel equal in playing ability and successful at performing skills at least part of the time. Occasional participation against superior players does, however, aid in increasing their skill.

However, some means of equalizing competition must be used. Many schemes are in use; such as age, height, weight, exponent system, selection of top players as captains, handicapping top teams, selecting players by classes, grading previous experience, using skill test scores, using classmates' rating of top players, etc. One or more of these schemes should be put into effect before team competition gets under way.

5. Absence of Instructor. The absence (some authorized adult should always be present) of the instructor should not cause bedlam to result or complete cessation of the planned program to occur. If the instructor has established an organizational plan that enables the students to function without the instructor being immediately present with them, it shows effective development of proper teacher-pupil class instructional relationship. This does not mean that the instructor retires to the sideline or to his office and lets the class run itself. It does help free the instructor to do individual teaching or to give instruction to part of the class membership at a time. If the instructor is called to the principal's office or to the telephone, the class should run itself. One older, top leader or skilled performer assigned to each 5 to 10 boys, who knows what is planned and is trained to carry out the details of the program regardless of the presence or absence of the instructor, is one way of planning effectively so that the class members are constantly learning, regardless of the whereabouts of the instructor. Such things as preparation for a discussion of a game, participation in skill tests, or trick exhibitions, etc., should be planned so that all students know what the objectives are. This aids in making this type of organization become a successful reality.

6. Consideration would be given to such student characteristics as maturity, state of school conditioning, home environment, personality (even of the class as a whole), degree of respect for the instructor, etc. How these characteristics may affect the way a group is organized may be illustrated by stating that the less mature (slow learning) students will respond best to demonstrations on how to perform a skill, and less to verbal explanation as contrasted with the more mature group. In some instances the former group will have to be told more often to refrain from participation in horseplay during the class period. Their attention can be focused effectively on one thing for less time than is true of the more mature group.

7. Enthusiasm is catching and so are certain other qualities, including an intense desire to learn. Likewise resistance to certain phases of the instructional program may be initiated by a few and half-heartedly accepted by many. Also, each class has its own total personality and such offers a challenge to the teacher. Usually, a good teacher is flexible enough and his material varied enough to meet this challenge successfully.

An instructor may have established a reputation for conducting such a fine course that the students are conditioned to respond to him in a favorable manner. A good rapport with the students in this instance is easier than normal to establish.

8. Establishing Class Standards and Rules. Establishment of the rules and regulations concerning the conduct of the class by the members of the class in cooperation with the instructor usually means that they will be obeyed by every student. Some of the typical types of rules and regulations that might be proposed are:

a. All students must wear clean and serviceable shoes and clothes. This rule should be enforced whether or not the clothes are uniform in design and color. The students should help the instructor decide what would be fair and just punishment for violators. Such a rule, however, must not be in conflict with any of the school's established policies.

b. The time allotted for dressing, showering, and changing clothes must be determined. Usually the time allotted is about 10 minutes for such procedures to be completed.

c. Employment of a quick, accurate, consistent method of roll taking that will not be complicated and difficult to administer is necessary. The roll taking method used should be one that any student leader could administer if called upon to do so. The type selected will depend upon the number of students, facilities, and their arrangement, type of absentee reports, etc.

Some roll taking methods that might be used are involved in such formations and procedures as a circle, with a prescribed number of students in it, squads, single or double lines, students standing and number painted on the floor, a slip with name on it turned in, a color and a number for each student, a place card with name on it held up, etc.

9. No Lulls in the Program. The students should not be given time nor opportunity to get into trouble. There must be a continuous learning environment provided for the students. Lulls in the program where students are forced to sit on the sidelines just watching for a long period of time provide the opportunity for students to do things other than to learn basketball skills.

10. Safety Factors. Safety factors must be taken into account when planning the program. The injury potential is high when a large class is practicing and playing basketball. Vigorous physical action under two adjacent baskets calls for good cooperation on the part of the students and alert supervision by the instructor to help to avoid the occurrence of injury. Boundary lines must be clearly defined and strictly adhered to by all of the participants. A quick method of recording and reporting to the proper office every injury that occurs must be established. Reasonable safety measures must be put into effect or else the teacher or school or both are liable for suit on the grounds of negligence.

It would be wise for the instructor to scrutinize the basketball court carefully each day before the class convenes in order to eliminate safety hazards. The following may cause injury to the students:

a. Loose basketball just lying on the floor as the students rush on to the court for play. It is better to have the basketballs placed in a large bag and then issued to the students after they arrive prepared for action.

b. Shirts or identification cloth strips lying on the floor in the path of the students may cause them to trip and fall to the floor.

c. Lack of protection mats placed against the wall under each basket may cause injuries.

d. Loose and/or wet boards which are a part of the floor of the court are a hazard.

FOUR-YEAR BASKETBALL PROGRAM FOR HIGH SCHOOL STUDENTS IN PHYSICAL EDUCATION CLASS

The program proposed here may be modified depending upon the number of students in each class and the extent of the facilities available.

I. *Freshman Year* (fundamentals emphasized)—A strong desire to play must be developed early in the students. The desired pattern of performance can be established easily with young players.
   A. Basic fundamentals should be taught early, such as:
      1. Dribbling.
      2. Catching.
      3. Shooting (set up, long, short shots of all kinds).
      4. Guarding.
      5. Stopping and starting.
      6. Foul shooting.
      7. Etc.
   B. Only bare essentials in each are presented.
   C. Single formations and simple drills are used.
   D. Short, frequent scrimmages are conducted.
   E. Teams are organized and scrimmages are held frequently.
   F. Pictures of known stars, especially in a series of pictures performing a specific skill are posted.
   G. A daily schedule of activities should be posted.
   H. Variety and increased complexity are the keys to holding the attention of the students.
   I. Several movies should be shown.
   J. Basic rules are discussed and interpreted.
   K. Many demonstrations are done by the instructor or a senior player.

II. *Sophomore Year* (Perfection of basics accented).

A. Charts are kept on abilities.
B. Ball handling, passing, and shooting is stressed.
C. The concept of real team and individual play is introduced.
D. Elementary strategy is presented.
E. Concepts of proper conditioning techniques are discussed.
F. Longer scrimmages are held.
G. All the ideas presented during the freshman year are reviewed.
H. More demonstrations are done by students, less by teacher.
I. Outside performers are invited to demonstrate moves or discuss ideas.
J. Jump shots and tip-ins are introduced.

III. *Junior Year* (Team play stressed).

A. Review all previous techniques and information.
B. Patterns of play with the use of one specific system are initiated.
C. More detail on fundamentals is presented.
D. Advanced skills such as fade-away, left handed hooks, etc., are attempted.
E. More movies are shown, as many as four or five.
F. Development of unorthodox shots is begun.
G. New rules are discussed.
H. Practice of clever ways of handling the ball is presented.
I. The class members are considered as if they were out for a team.

IV. *Senior Year* (High level skills and team play blended).

A. Zone and man-to-man systems of play are used.
B. Strategy is tried out.
C. Moves such as eluding a guard, cutting by the post, etc., are attempted.
D. Varsity skill by the students is expected (but at a low level).
E. Top players are selected from the class to scrimmage against the varsity players.
F. It is suggested to the students that they form into units and play as teams on the outside of school.
G. The tempo of the class practice is fast and rapid.
H. Evaluation of the varsity games is made. Reports are presented.
I. The boys are given a chance to organize their own practice sessions and conduct classes.
J. Senior students are asked to assist in the teaching of underclassmen.
K. Interested class members are asked to help scout opponents of the varsity team.

Major Differences Between International and Collegiate Basketball Rules*

It is believed that almost all of the rules mentioned here will be adopted by all countries within a very few years. In fact all but two major countries now utilize the international rules. At the present time in the United States, there are collegiate rules, international amateur federation rules (for men and women when engaging in international competition), two sets of professional rules, AAU-DGWS rules for girls and women, women's collegiate rules, and more than one set of rules for high school girls (however, many are using the AAU-DGWS or high school federation rules.) Some differences are:

1. There is a 30-second clock or device which is put in operation when a team gains possession of the ball and lasts until a try for goal is made; thus allowing only 30 seconds to elapse before a shot must be attempted.
2. The act of "dunking" the ball is considered to be legal.
3. Both technical and personal fouls are included together in the total five fouls which eliminate a player from the game.
4. A player is allowed only 5 seconds in which to shoot a free throw.
5. The 3-second rule is in effect in a somewhat different manner in addition to the collegiate rules, that is, it also applies during out-of-bounds conditions and starts when the player has possession of the ball, not after it is thrown in from out-of-bounds.
6. A substitution may be made only by the team in possession of the ball when the clock is stopped by a violation. However, once a substitution is made by the eligible team, the other team may also make a substitution.
7. The 3-second lane is wider than in collegiate rules.
8. If a player, fouled in the act of shooting, scores, he is not awarded any foul shots but if he misses the field goal attempt he receives two free throws.
9. If a player is awarded two free shots, his team has the option of electing to put the ball into play from out-of-bounds at the middle of the nearest side line or to shoot the free throws.
10. Technical fouls are infractions that are treated very much like personal fouls in many instances. Those considered infractions carry a penalty of two free throws, others may be for one free throw.
11. Time-outs are called only by the coach with each team being allowed only two per half.
12. Team members are numbered on the back and front from 4 to 15.

*See AAU Official Handbook 1972–74 Basketball pp. 50–51, pp. 56–84 and 85–111.

13. Somewhat the same rules apply in relation to an offensive or defensive player touching the ball during its downward flight toward the basket when the ball is above the level of the basket, that is, it is illegal to do so. In international rules the restriction also applies to a pass.

14. The officials do not handle the ball on the throw-ons after violations.

15. Players are not permitted to throw a ball against an opponent and maintain control of it.

16. After a successful free throw or field goal is the only time a team makes a throw-in from the end of the court.

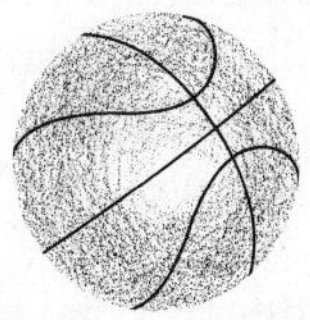

Glossary

Back court: That half of the playing court in which the opponents conduct their offensive maneuvers.

Backdoor: When an offensive player cuts toward the basket and behind the opposing defender in order to receive a pass from a teammate. The term is often used synonymously with the term "blind pig."

Baseline: The line marking the ends (lengthwise) of the playing surface.

Blind Pig: Used interchangeably with the term "backdoor."

Clear out: Usually refers to an offensive maneuver in which players vacate a portion of the floor so as to isolate one offensive and one defensive player. The offensive player may then attempt to score against his opponent and the opponent has no teammates that are close enough to come to his aid.

Cue defense: Refers to a defense that changes strategy on the basis of some predetermined signal.

Cut: An accelerated, quick movement on the part of an offensive player that is directed toward the basket. Most often the cut is made around a teammate in an attempt to screen off the defensive player.

Front court: That half of the playing court in which the team conducts its offensive maneuvers.

Give and go: Refers to an offensive maneuver in which a player passes to a teammate and breaks for the basket expecting to receive a quick return pass.

Jump or held ball: Occurs when the referee halts play because two opposing players have joint possession of the ball. The two players then proceed to jump at the nearest jump ball area in order to determine possession of the ball.

Key: Refers to the semi-circle area that begins at the free throw line and ends the half-court line.

Lane: Refers to the 12 foot wide and 18 foot 10 inch long area from the free throw line to the baseline. An offensive player may not stay in this area for longer than three seconds at a time.

Outlet Pass: Refers to the first pass made after a successful defensive rebound has been made.

Pick and roll: Refers to an offensive maneuver in which a player screens for a teammate who has the ball and then after the screen is completed, executes a reverse roll movement and breaks toward the basket expecting to receive a return pass from his teammate.

Post or pivot man: The two terms are interchangeable and refer to the offensive center of a team.

Scissors: Same as split.

Split: Refers to an offensive crisscross maneuver in which two players cut by on opposite sides of a teammate who has the ball. Synonymous with the term scissors.

Strong side: Refers to the side of the court (divided lengthwise) in which the ball is located.

Switch: A defensive maneuver in which two defenders exchange defensive responsibilities by exchanging the men they are guarding. Occurs most frequently during a screening situation in which one of the defenders can no longer guard his man because of the screen.

Tip: Refers to the momentary catching and pushing movement made by the offensive rebounder in an attempt to score from an offensive rebound while he is still in the air.

Trap: A defensive maneuver in which two defenders attempt to stop an offensive dribbler and prevent him from making a successful pass.

Weak side: Refers to the side of the court (divided lengthwise) opposite to the strong side.

Wing: A high forward offensive position.

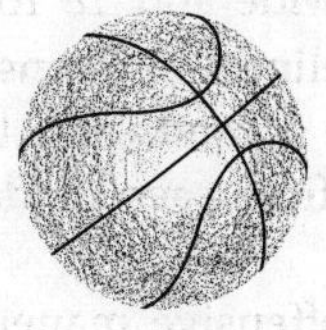

Sample Diagrams of Team Offenses

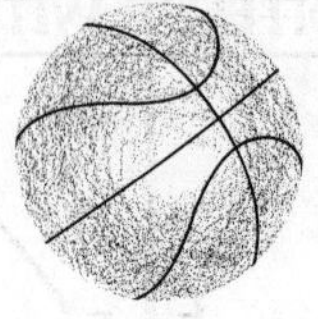

Sample Diagrams of Team Offenses

C	Center
P	Post or Pivot
F	Forward
G	Guard
W	Wing
L	Left or Low
R	Right
H	High
M	Middle

EXAMPLES

LG	Left Guard	HP	High Post
RW	Right Wing	LP	Low Post
LLP	Left Low Post	MG	Middle Guard

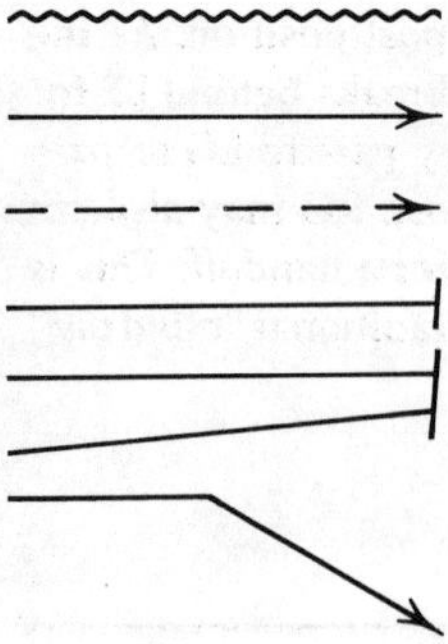

(wavy line) . . . Dribble

(solid line with arrow) . . . Player Movement Without Possession of the Ball

(dashed line with arrow) . . . Pass

(line ending in a crossbar) . . . Screen

(two lines ending in one crossbar) . . . Double Screen

(line that bends, ending in an arrow) . . . Cut

SINGLE POST OFFENSE WITH A LOW POST

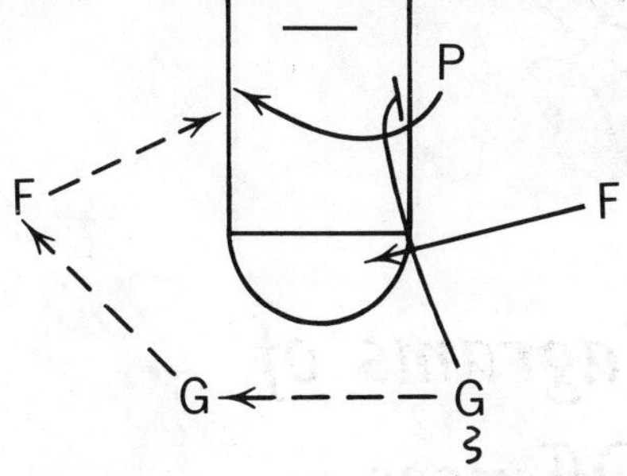

This offense is often used to take advantage of the scoring potential of a very tall center. In this play RG passes to LG. RG then cuts down the lane as LG passes to LF. RF cuts to the lane behind RG's cut. RG then screens for P who breaks across the lane into a low post position. LF may pass the ball either to RF or P.

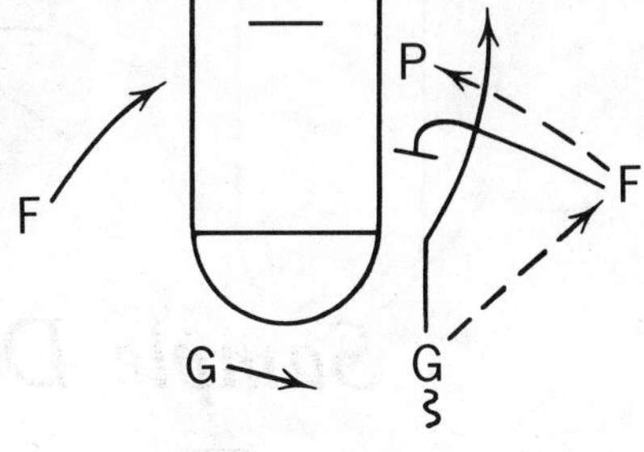

In this play RG passes the ball to RF. RF passes to P in the low post. RF and RG then scissor off the low post with RF having the option of stopping his cut to screen for RG or to continue on toward the basket.

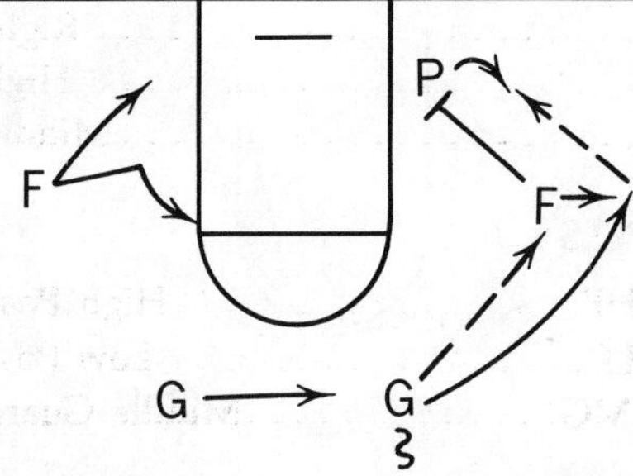

In this play RG passes to RF and cuts to his outside for a return handoff. RF then cuts toward the basket and sets a screen for P. LF can either break to a weakside rebounding position or break to a high post position.

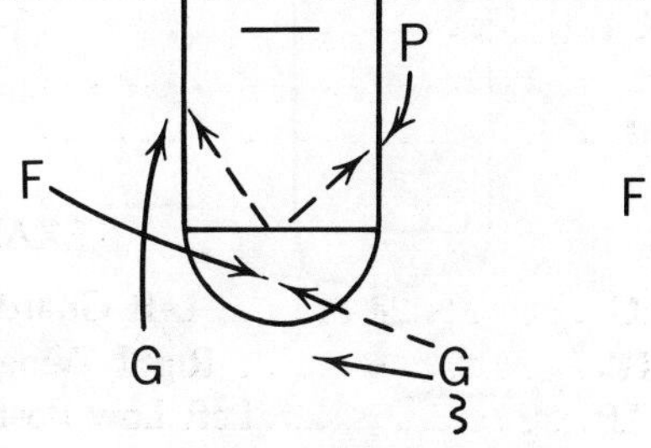

In this play RG passes to LF who has moved to a high post position. As the pass is made LG breaks behind LF for the basket. LF may pass to LG or pass to P in the low post. RG may also cut off the high post for a handoff. This is a variation of the traditional "blind pig" play.

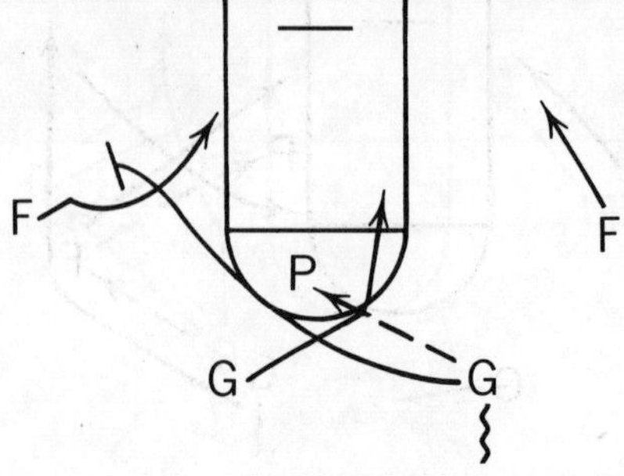

In using this offense the pivot man plays with his back to the basket along the free throw line. In this play RG passes to P. LG and RG then scissor off P with RG going first and continuing to screen for LF who cuts off the screen toward the basket.

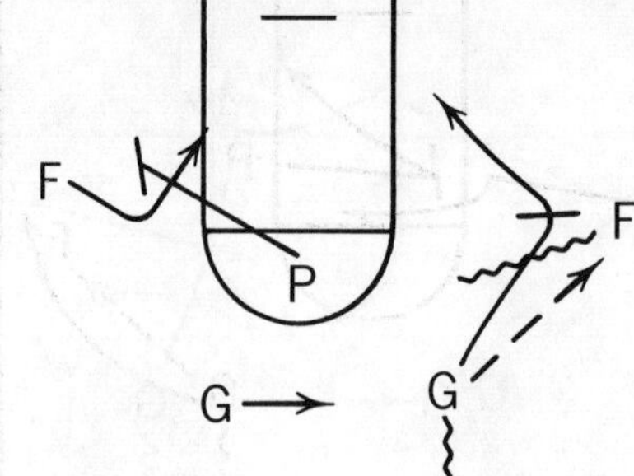

In this play RG passes to F. RG then sets an inside screen for F. F dribbles by the screen and RG rolls to the basket. As the screen is set, P screens opposite for LF who cuts sharply down the lane toward the basket.

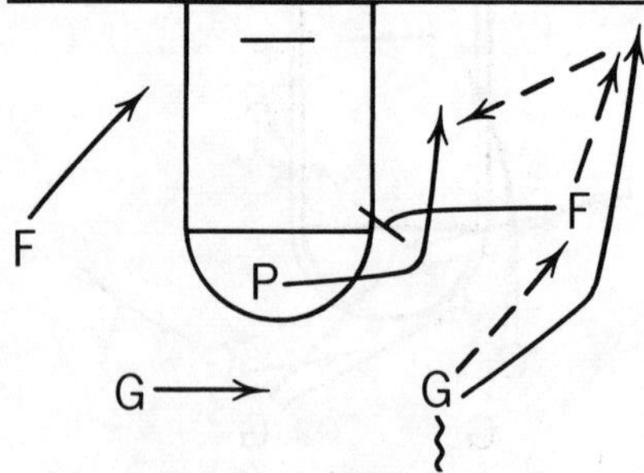

In this play RG passes to RF and cuts around him toward the corner. RF passes to RG in the corner. RF then sets a screen for P who cuts down the lane.

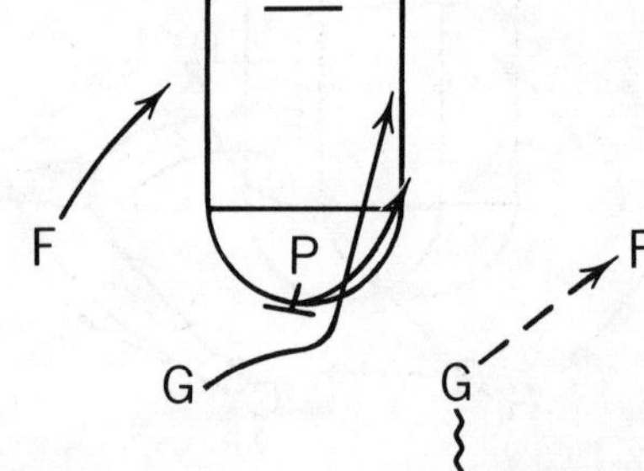

In this play RG passes to RF. P sets a screen for LG who cuts sharply down the lane. P rolls from the screen to a medium high post on the strong side.

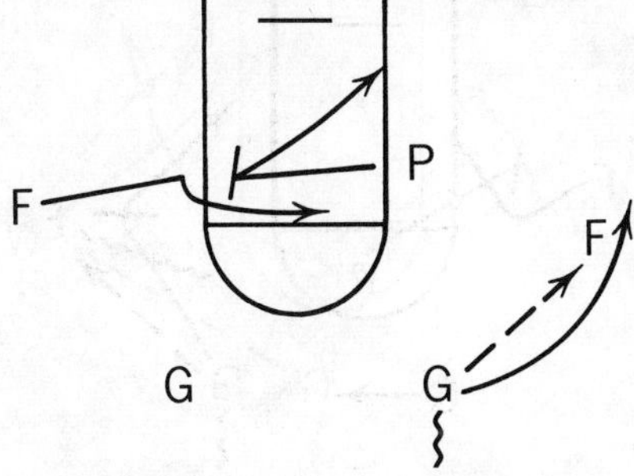

In using this offense the pivot man operates about half way between the free throw line and the basket. In this play RG passes to RF and cuts to his outside. P screens opposite for LF who cuts into the lane.

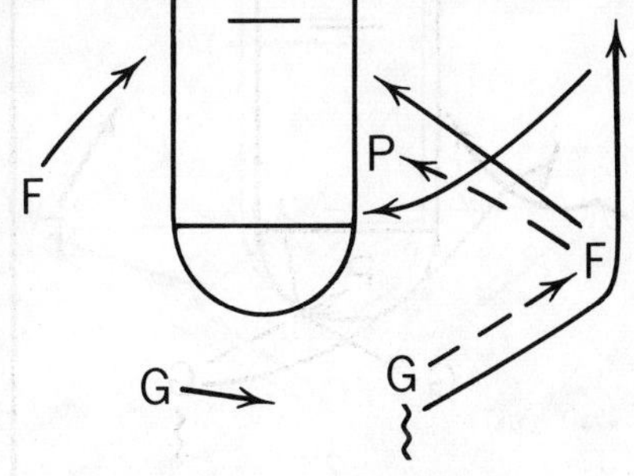

In this play RG passes to RF and cuts around him toward the corner. RF passes to P. RF and RG then scissor off P.

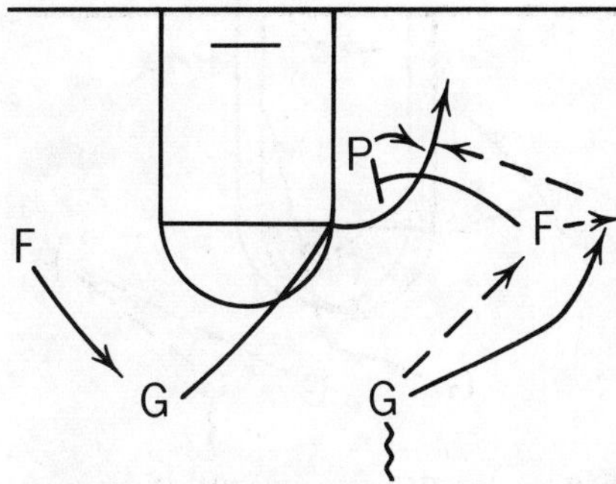

In this play G passes to RF and cuts around him getting a return pass. RF then screens for P who gets the pass from RG. RG and LG then scissor off P. LF moves so as to maintain floor balance.

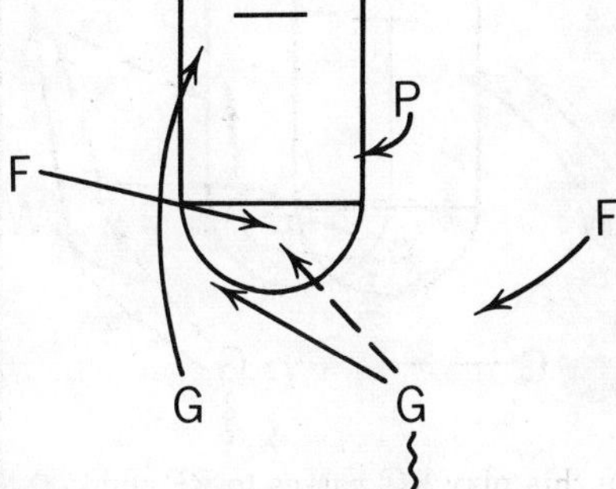

In this play RG passes to LF who cuts into a high post position. LG then cuts behind LF looking for a lob or bounce pass near the basket. This is sometimes called the "blind pig" play.

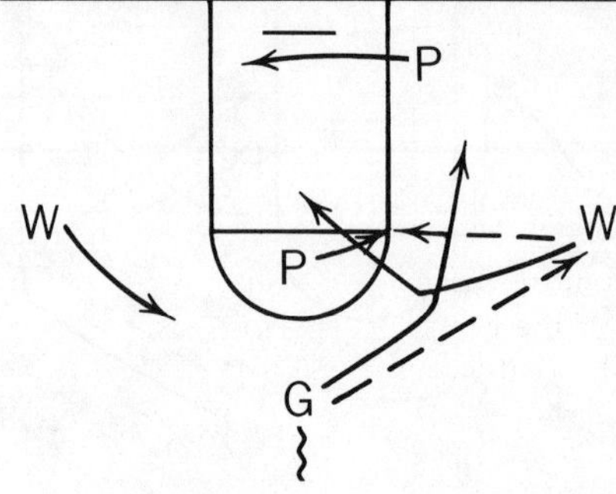

This offense utilizes a high post and a low post, two wing men, and a guard. In this basic play, G passes to RW. RW passes to HP who has moved to a high side post. RW and G then scissor off HP.

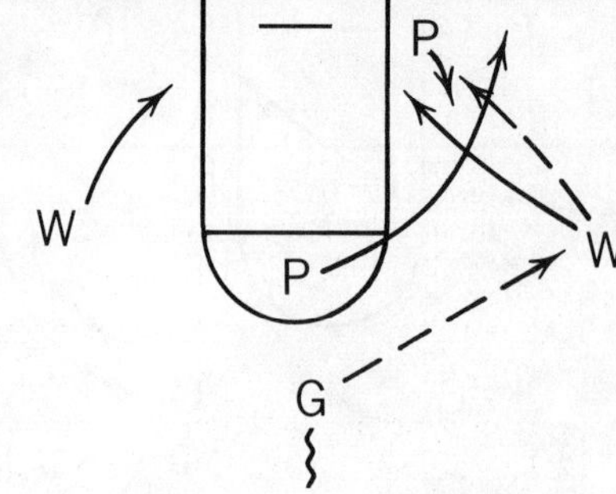

In this basic play G passes to RW. RW passes to LP. RW and HP then scissor off LP. LW rebounds on the weakside, while G maintains floor balance.

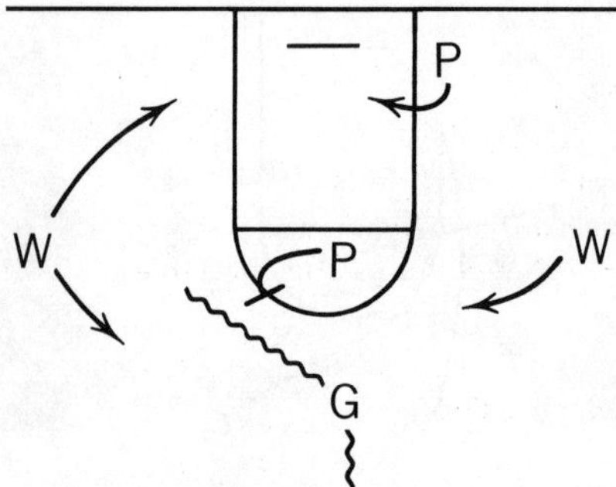

In this play HP sets a screen for G. LW can either attempt to backdoor his opponent or he can move into an outside weave with G and RW.

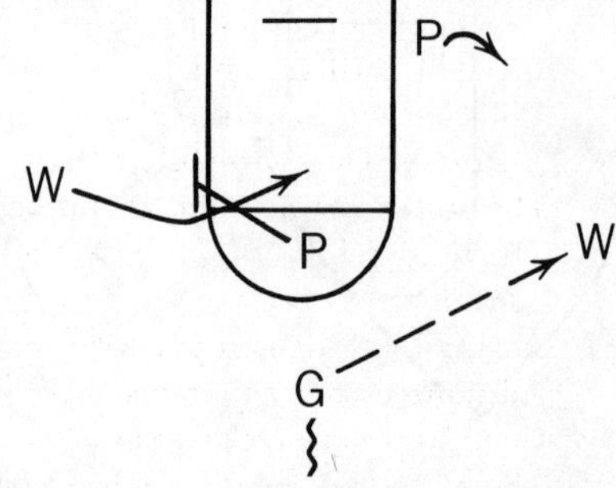

In this play G passes to RW. HP screens opposite for LW who cuts down the lane. LP sets up in a strong side low post. RW could pass to LP and cut by him, or he could try to hit LW breaking down the lane.

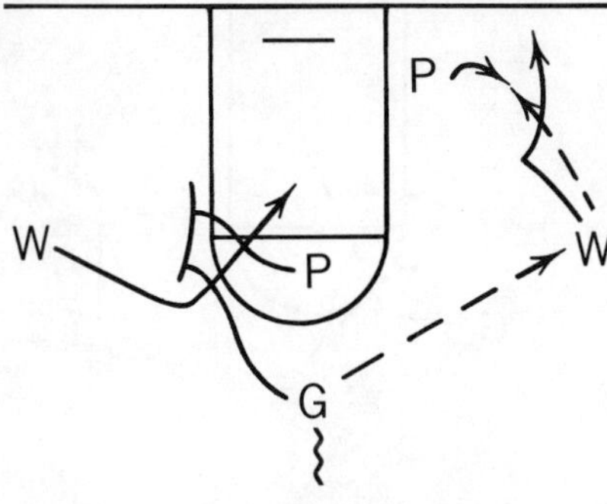

In this play G passes to RW. G and HP then set a double screen for LW. LP moves out to a wide low post. RW passes to LP and cuts to his outside. LP can handoff to RW or try to hit LW breaking down the lane.

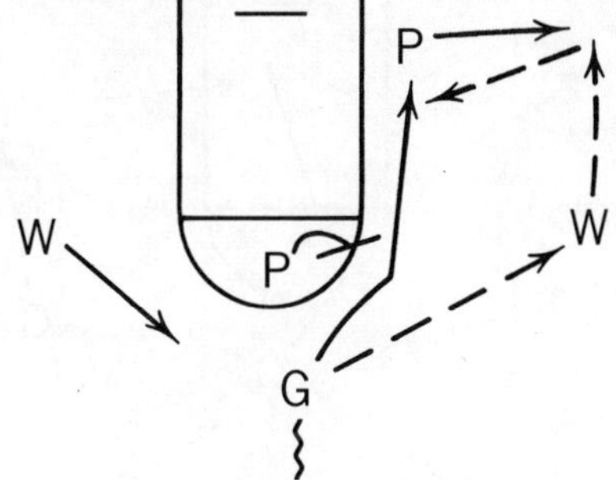

In this play G passes to RW. LP moves out to a wide low post. RW passes to LP. HP sets a screen for G who breaks down the lane. LP attempts to hit G on his break. LW moves toward center court to establish floor balance.

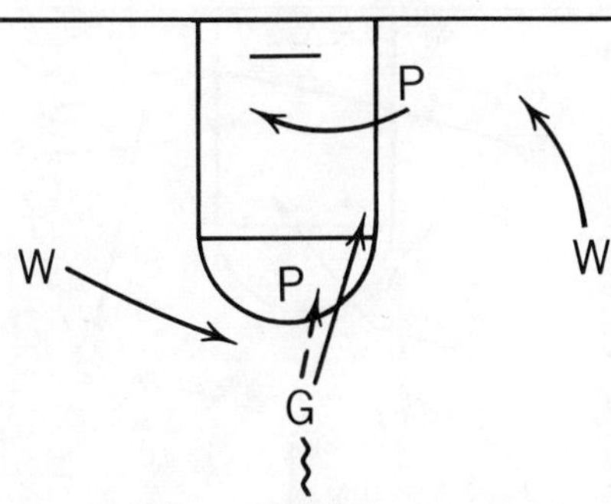

In this play G passes to HP. As G cuts off HP, RW attempts to backdoor his opponent. LP moves across the lane to a low post position, and LW cuts on the high side of HP.

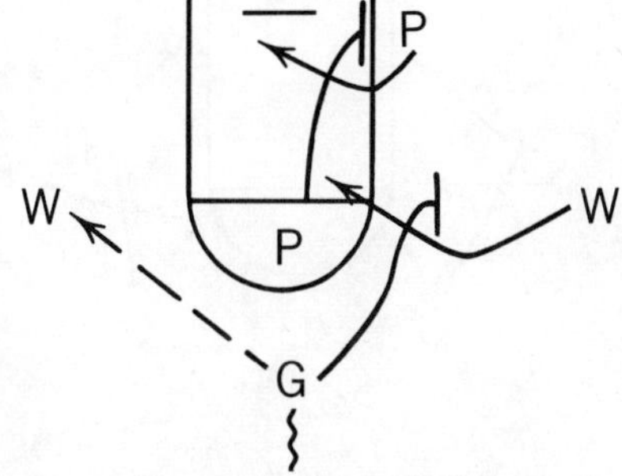

In this play G passes to LW. G and HP then set simultaneous screens for RW and LP. LW attempts to hit either cutter with the ball.

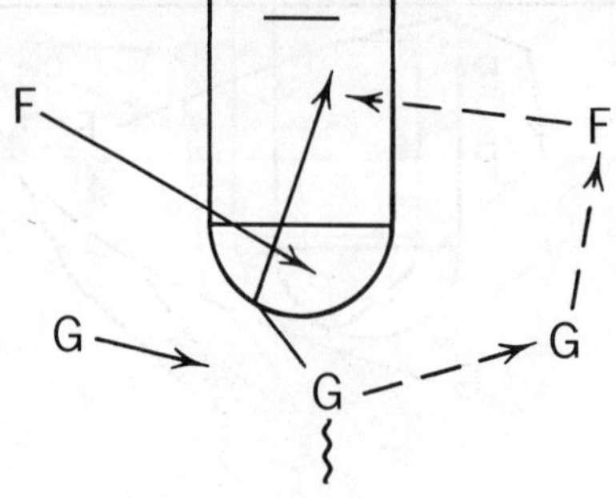

This offense is often utilized when the team lacks a big pivot man, but has players who are fairly mobile and of equal size. In this play MG passes to RG. RG passes to RW. While this pass is made LW breaks to a high post position. MG breaks behind this post in an attempt to screen off his man. RW attempts to pass to MG close to the basket.

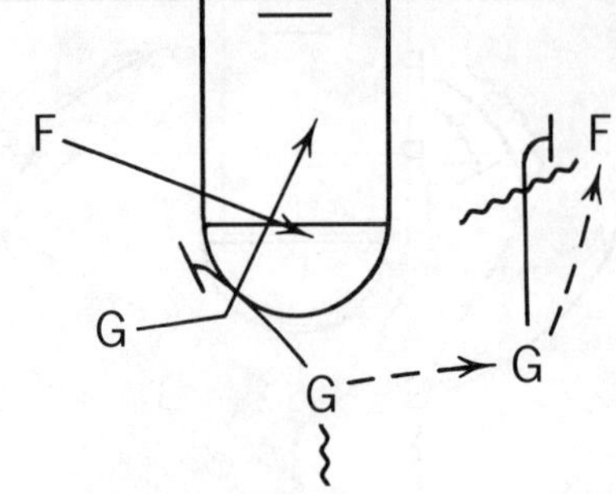

In this play MG passes to RG and then screens opposite for LG. RG passes to RF and then sets an inside screen for him. RF dribbles off the screen looking for LG breaking down the lane or LF breaking to a high post position.

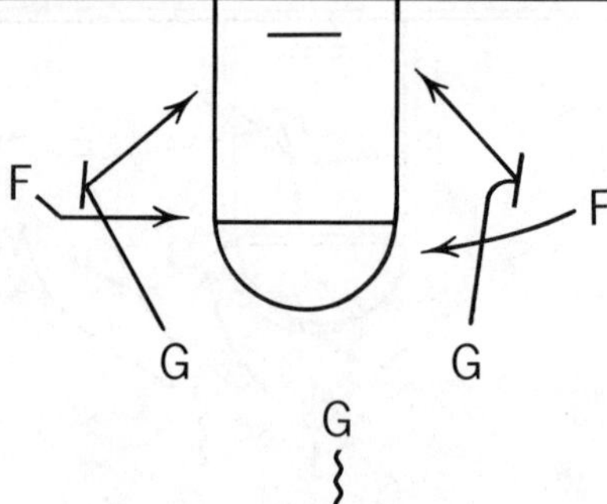

In this play LG screens for LF and RG screens for RF as MG brings the ball into the scoring area. After the screen is completed LG and RG roll toward the basket making sure not to cross the lane. MG may pass to either F.

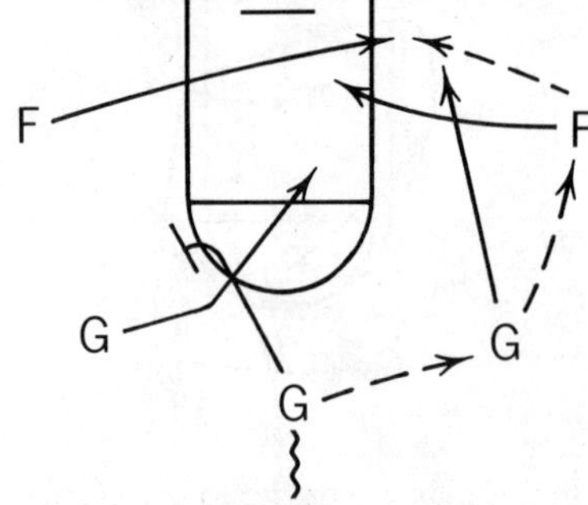

In this play MG passes to RG and moves to screen for LG. RG passes to RF. While this pass is made LF is breaking across the lane into a low post position. RF passes to LF. RF and RG scissor off the low post.

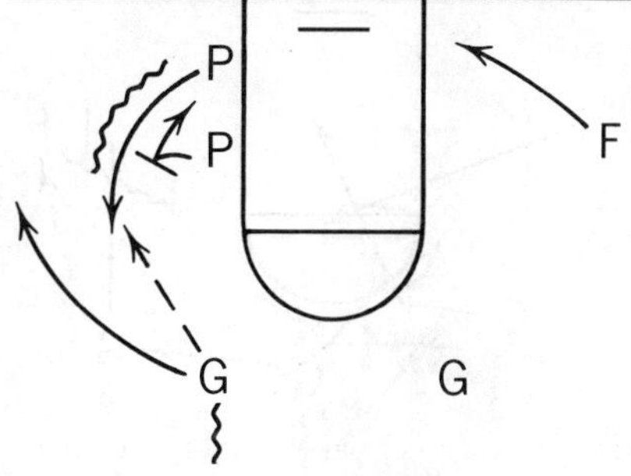

This offense was used by Coach Ed Jucker while he was at Cincinnati University. It utilizes two pivot men in a close tandem on one side of the lane. In this basic play the low P breaks around the high P to receive a pass from LG. High P then screens for LP. This screen can be an inside or outside screen. LP moves by the screen and HP rolls toward the basket.

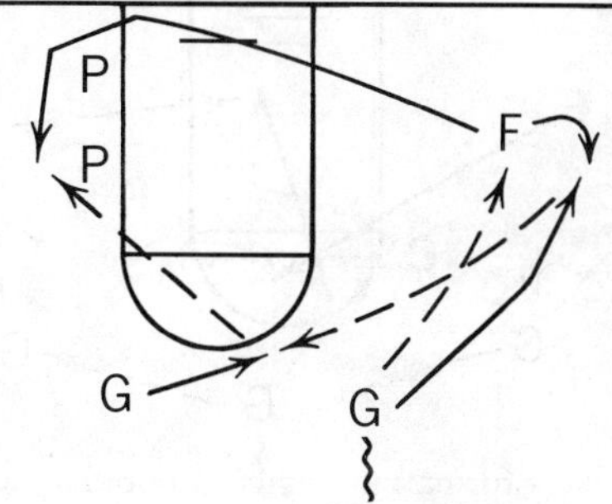

In this play LG passes to F who has broken behind a double screen set by the high and low P.

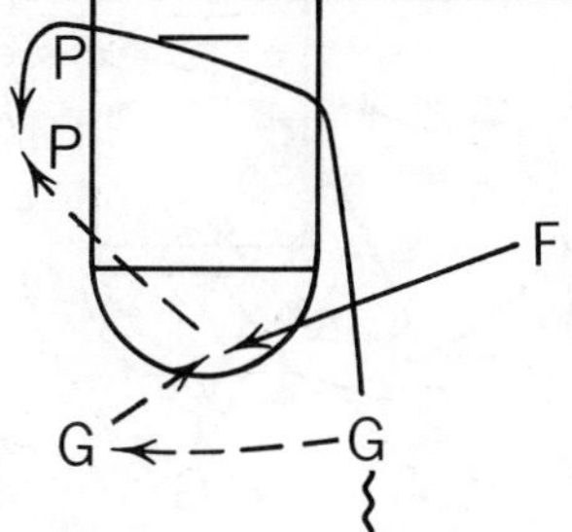

In this play RG passes to LG. LG passes to F who has broken to a high post position. RG breaks behind F and moves across the lane behind the double screen set by high P and low P.

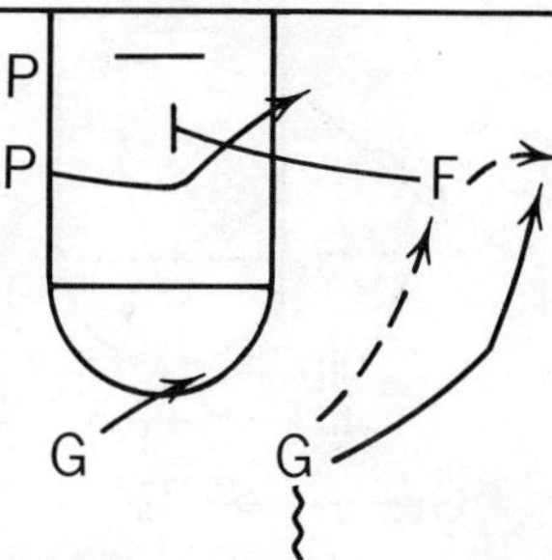

In this play RG passes to F and cuts to his outside for a return handoff. F then moves to screen for high P or low P who cuts across the lane to a low post position on the other side.

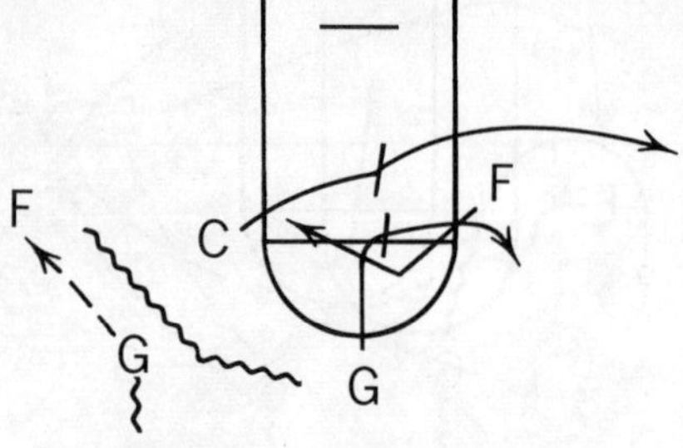

This formation depicts a popular continuity offense that involves a great deal of cutting and screening. It is sometimes called the Auburn Shuffle or the Drake Shuffle. The offense requires that players take precise positions on the floor. In this play LG passes to LF. RG and C set a double screen for RF. Notice that at the end of the movement the five players have taken up positions that are the "mirror" positions of the ones in which they started. They have "turned over" the offense.

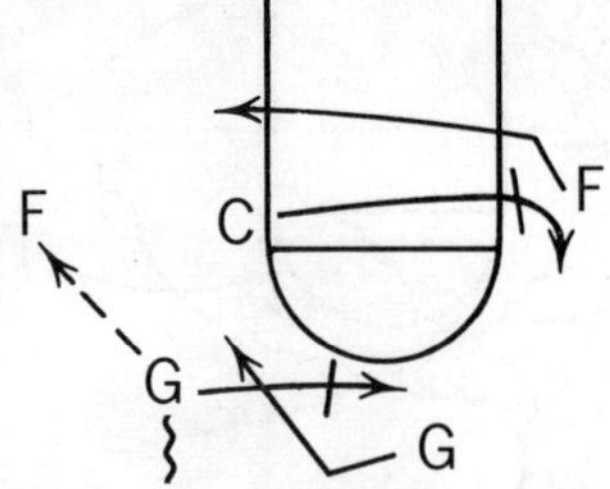

In this play LG passes to LF and then screens for RG who cuts toward LF. C screens opposite for RF. After the movements are completed the five original positions on the floor are again filled, but by different players with the exception of LF.

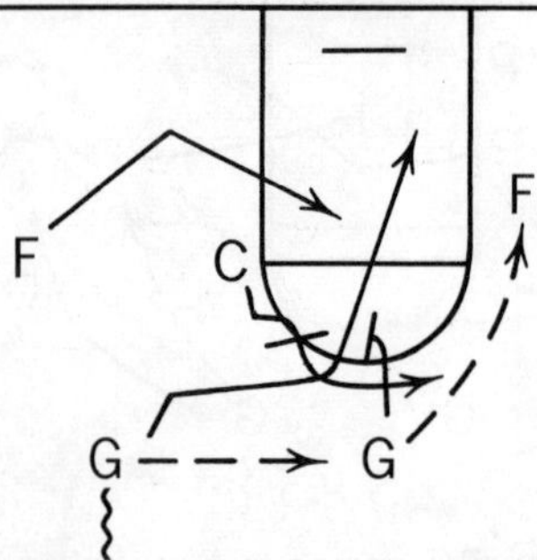

In this play LG passes to RG. RG passes to RF. LG cuts past a screen set by C. RG then screens for C who breaks to the top of the key. LF has faked a break to the basket and cut back toward the center of the lane. RF may pass to LG, C, or LF.

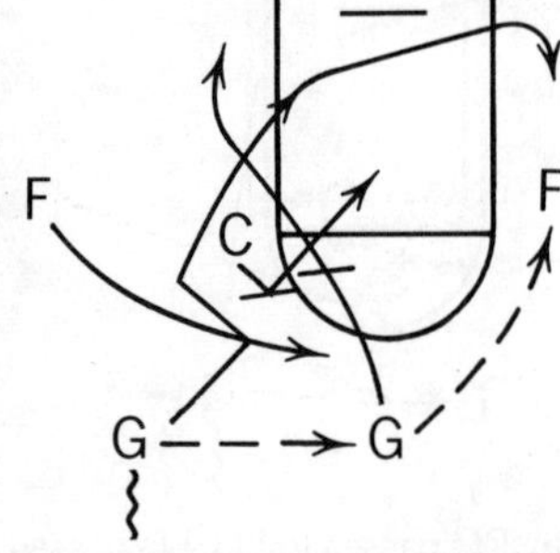

In this play LG passes to RG. RG passes to RF. RG and C set a double screen. LG cuts behind the screen and across the lane. LF cuts on top of the screen. C and RG both roll from the screen with C being the intended receiver of the pass from RF.

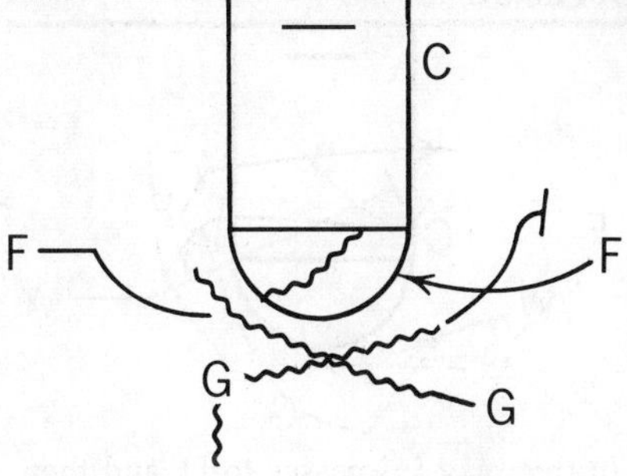

This is a four man weave designed to create an opening for a player to drive toward the basket or take a jump shot from the free throw line area. LG initiates the weave and moves to screen for RF after he had handed off the ball to RG.

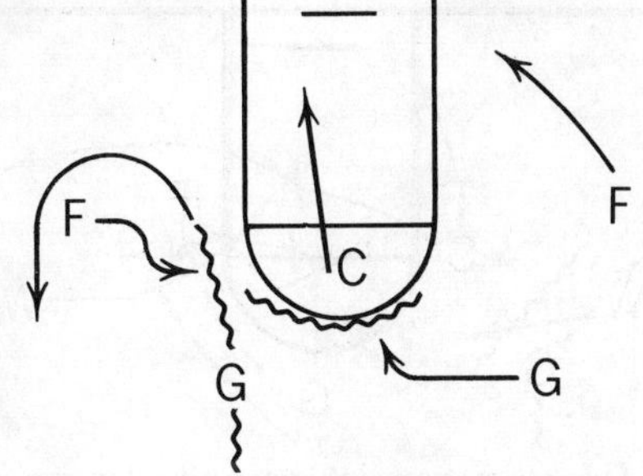

In this weave pattern the center plays in a high pivot position and screens for RG who is the third man in the weave.

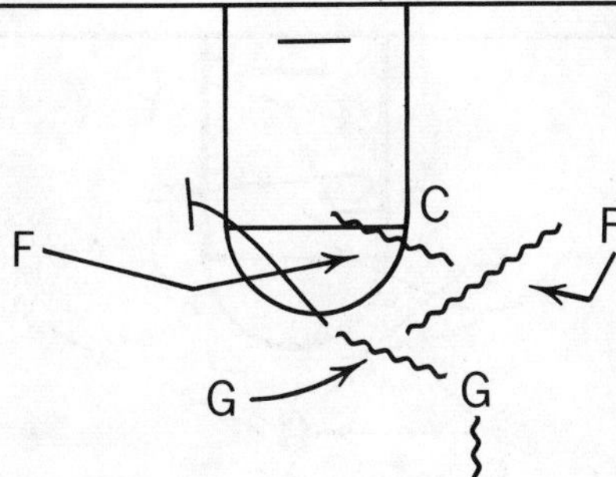

This is the same four man weave as shown directly above but it is initiated to the opposite side. Notice also that C is placed in a higher post position and could be utilized as a screener by LF who is the fourth man in the weave.

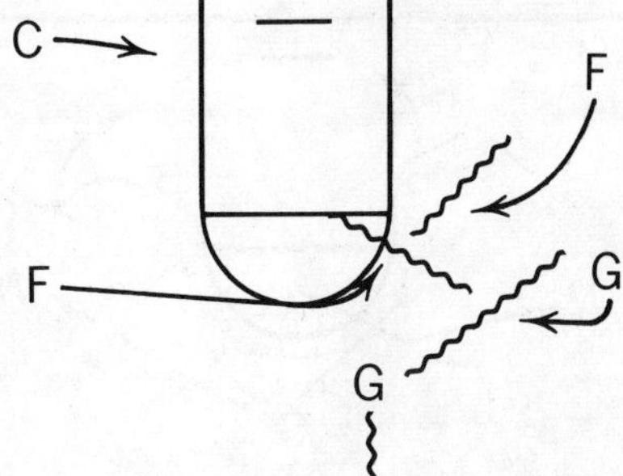

This is a five man weave with no pivot man. Notice how G who initiates the weave loops back to provide defensive balance and also to be able to become a part of the weave again.

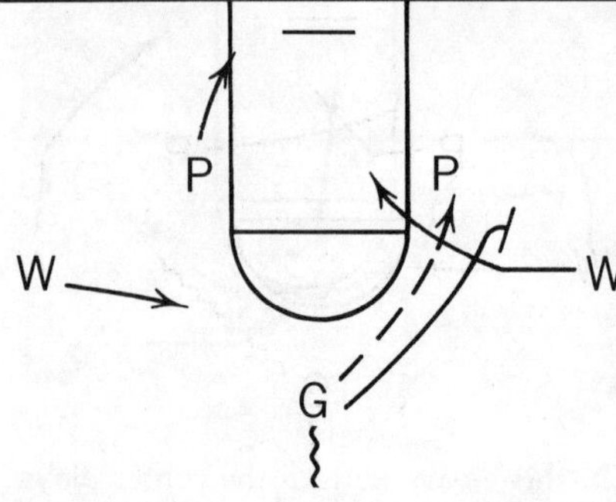

This offense utilizes two high post men, two wing men, and one guard. The basic positioning of the players makes this double cut one of the best scoring plays to use in this type of offense. Notice how G screens for W, who is the second cutter.

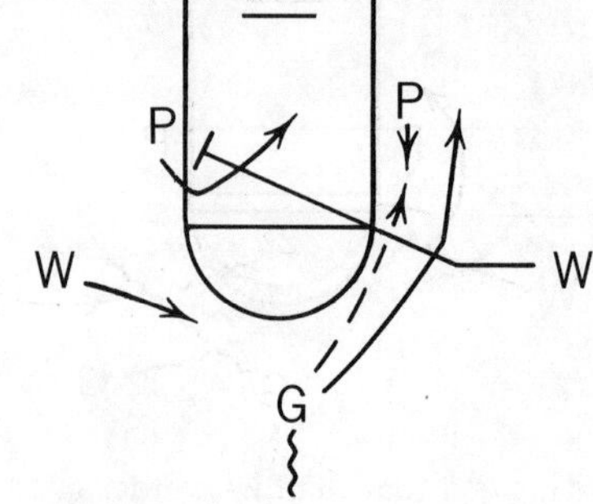

In this play, RW initiates the play by cutting through to screen for the LP who cuts sharply to the basket. G then passes to RP and cuts sharply by him. RP can pass to LP, give the ball back to G for the drive or jump shot, or he can keep the ball himself and attempt his own scoring movements.

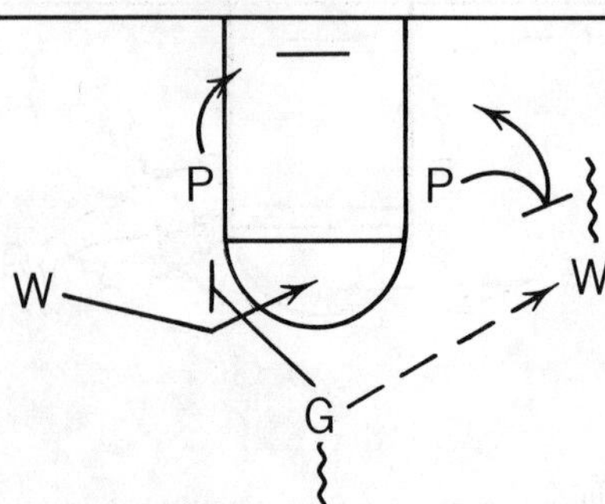

G initiates this play by passing to RW. G then screens on the opposite side for LW who cuts to the free throw line. RP sets a screen for RW. RW can pass to LW, or he can work the pick and roll play with RP.

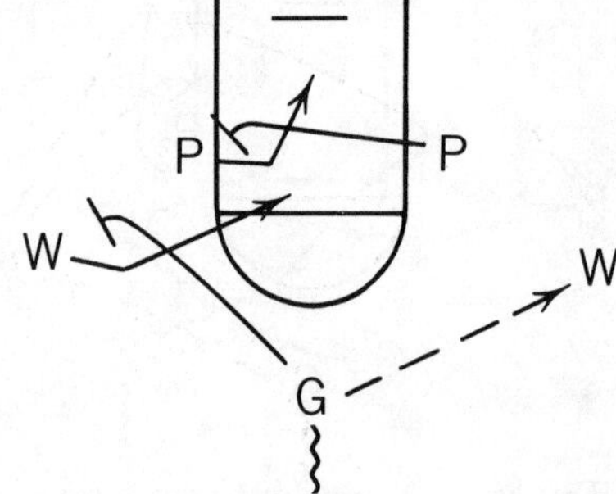

G initiates this play by passing to RW. G then screens on the opposite side for LW and RP also screens to the opposite side for LP. RW can pass to either cutter or he can initiate his own offensive movements because his side of the floor has been cleared out.

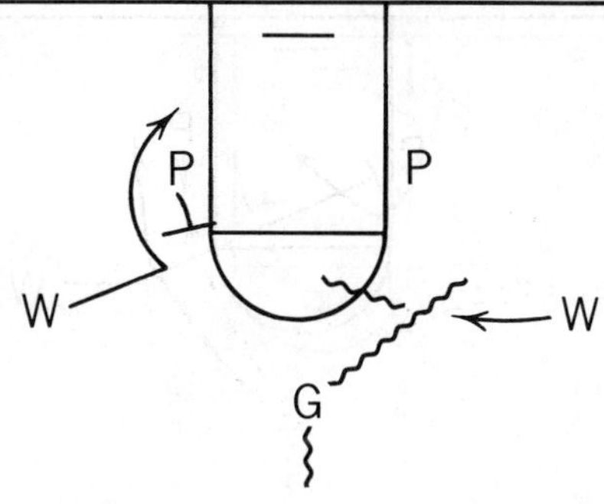

In this play G starts the three man outside weave with RW, but LW, who also has the option of continuing the weave, breaks behind LP in an attempt to "backdoor" his defensive opponent.

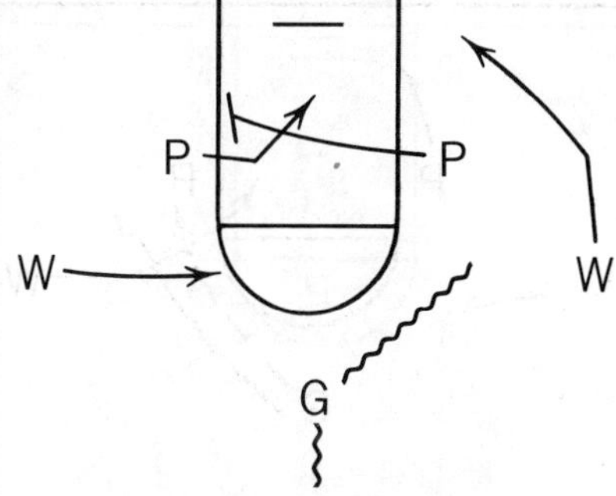

In this play G dribbles toward RW who clears out the right side of the floor in an attempt to backdoor his opponent. RP screens to the opposite side for LP who cuts toward the basket. LW moves toward the center court to maintain floor balance.

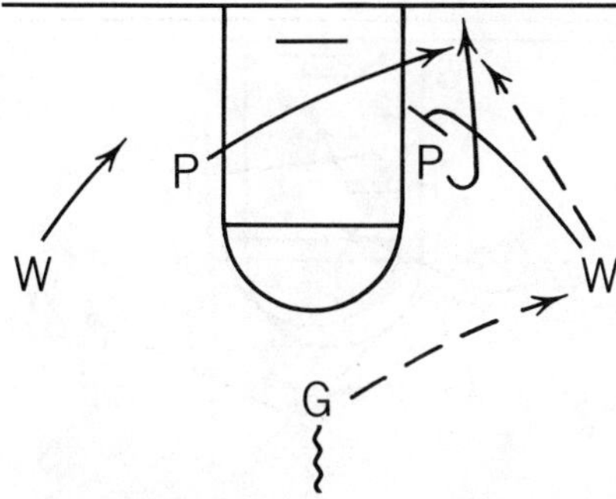

In this play G passes to RW. RW passes to LP who has cut across to set up a low post. RW then moves toward the basket as if to cut off the low post but instead sets a screen for RP who cuts off the screen and low post.

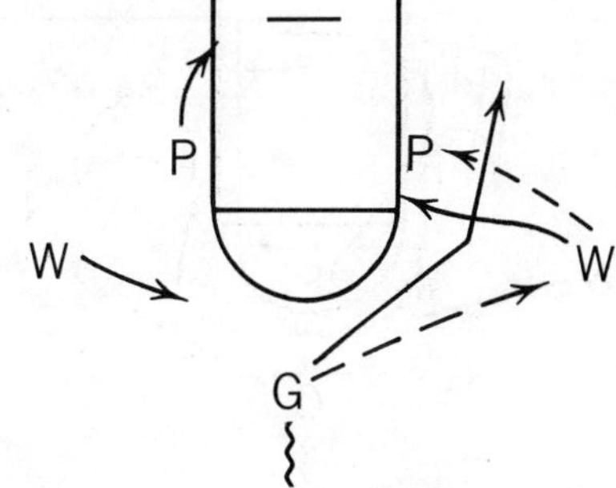

In this play G passes to RW. RW passes to RP. RW and G then scissor off RP. RW can actually cut for the basket or he can screen for G who is the second man on the cut. LP moves for a rebounding position, while LW establishes floor balance.

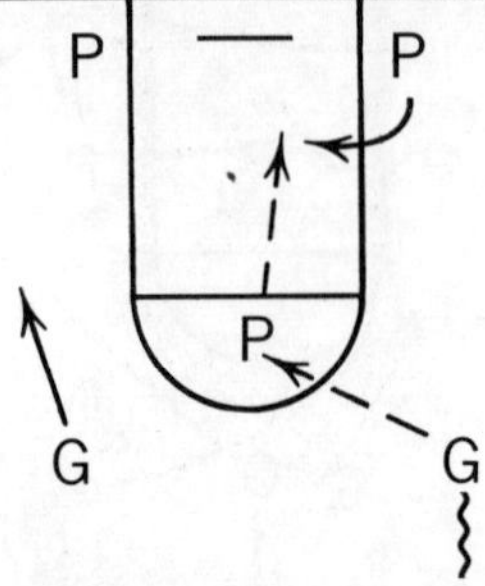

This offense is often utilized when a team has three tall players who perform best close to the basket. Coach Tex Winter used a triple post offense while he was at Kansas State University. In this play RG passes to HP. HP immediately turns and attempts to pass to one of the LP's breaking into the lane.

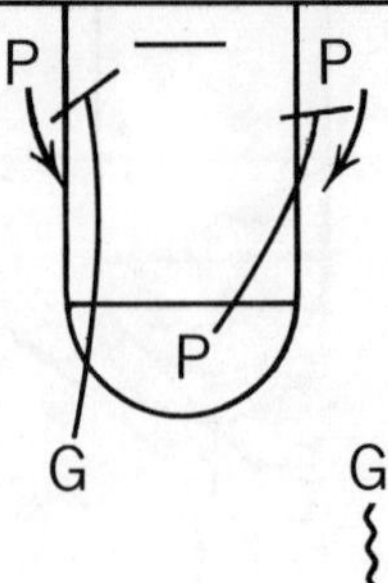

In this play a double screening situation is set up as RG brings the ball into the scoring area. LG moves straight down the lane to screen for LLP and HP rolls down the other side of the lane to screen for RLP. RG may pass to either of the LP's.

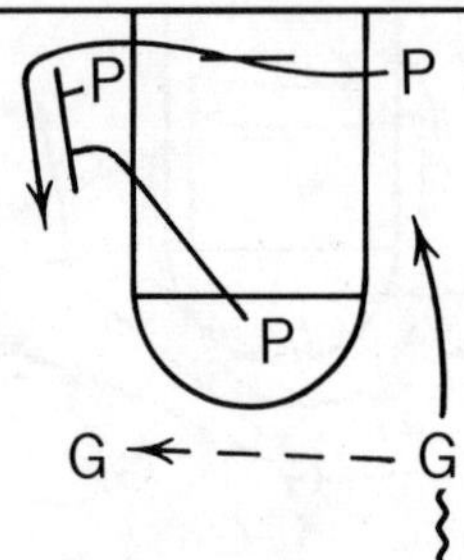

In this play RG passes to LG. HP moves down the left side of the lane to set a double screen with LLP. RLP breaks behind the double screen. As he does this, RG attempts to backdoor his opponent. LG can either pass to RLP or he can attempt to make a lob pass to RG.

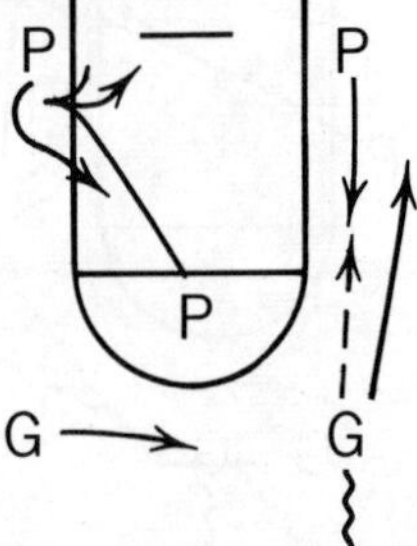

In this play RG passes to RLP who has broken up to a medium post position. As this pass is made HP moves to screen for LLP. RG breaks by RLP looking for the return pass. LLP breaks around the screen into the lane looking for the pass so he can attempt the short shot.

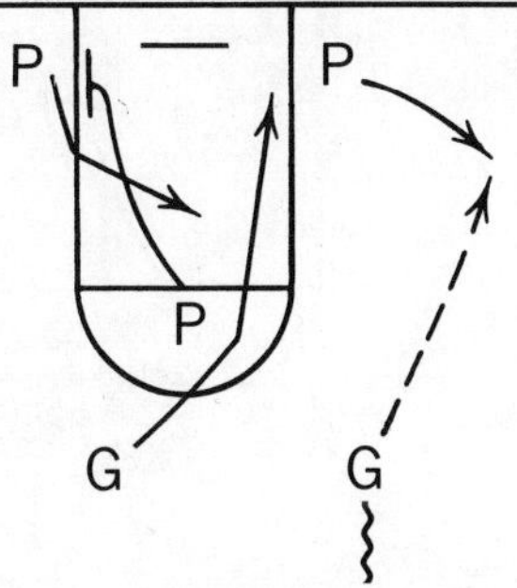

In this play RG passes to RLP who has moved to a wing position. LG attempts to screen his man by breaking past HP. After LG has made his cut HP rolls opposite to screen for LLP who cuts into the lane.

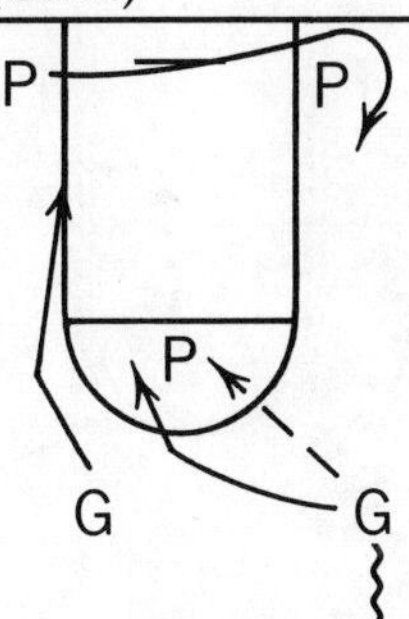

In this play RG passes to HP. LG attempts to backdoor his man. LLP breaks across the lane and behind RLP in an attempt to screen his man. HP may pass to LG, handoff to RG breaking by the high post, or he may pass to LLP.

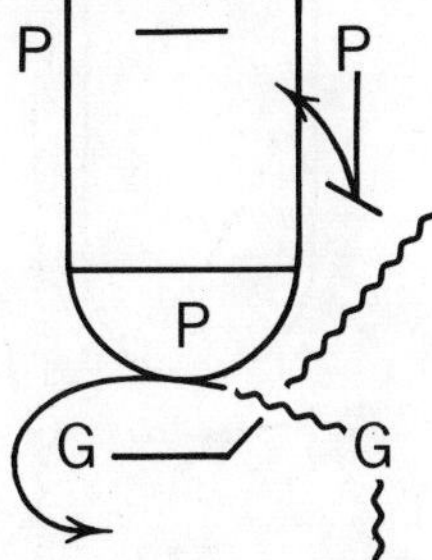

In this play RG starts a weave maneuver with LG. LG continues on to take advantage of the pick and roll situation setup by RLP.

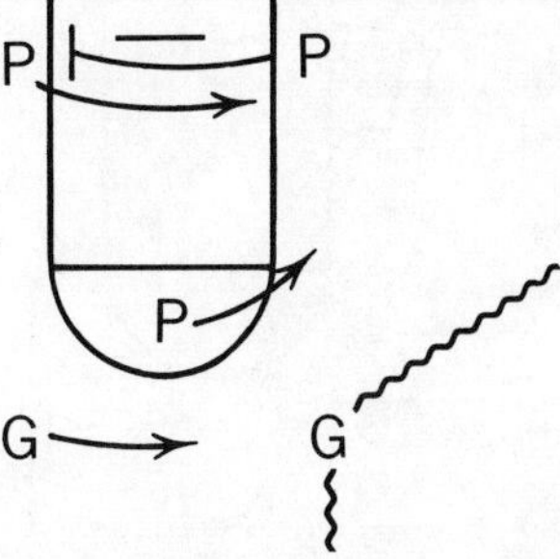

In this play RG dribbles into a swing position. RLP moves across the lane to screen for LLP. RG may pass to HP who has broken to a side post position or to LLP who has broken to a low post position.

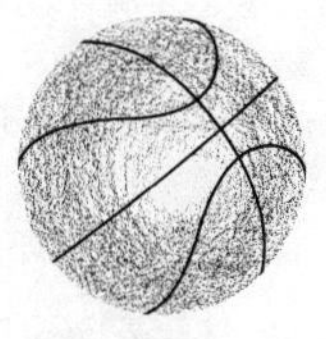

Sample Diagrams of Team Defenses

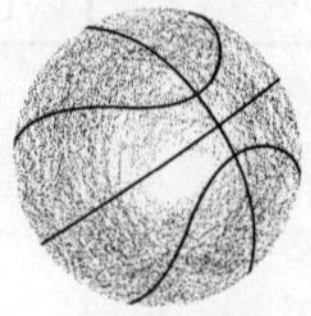

Sample Diagrams of Team Defenses

C . . . . Center
P . . . . Post
F . . . . Forward
G . . . . Guard
W . . . . Wing
L . . . . Left or Low
R . . . . Right
H . . . . High
M . . . . Middle

EXAMPLES

LG . . . . Left Guard
RW . . . . Right Wing
LLP . . . . Left Low Post
HP . . . . High Post
LP . . . . Low Post
MG . . . . Middle Guard

(wavy line) . . . . Dribble
(solid arrow) . . . Player Movement Without Possession of the Ball
(dashed arrow) . . . . Pass
(line ending in bar) . . . . Screen
(two lines ending in bar) . . . . Double Screen
(angled arrow) . . . . Cut

DEFENSE AGAINST THE TWO ON TWO SCREENING SITUATIONS

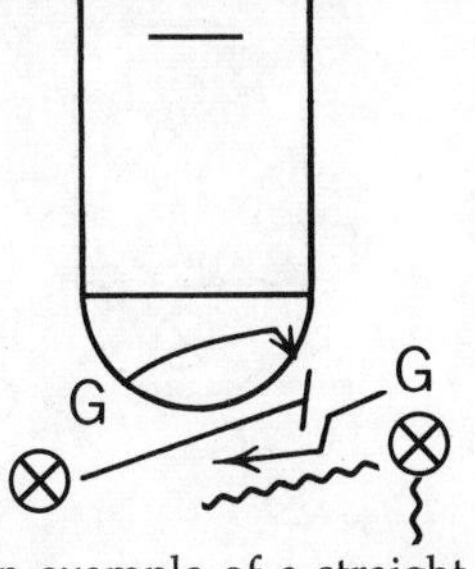

This is an example of a straight man-to-man defense that is being played very aggressively. Notice that the defensive player guarding the dribbler steps up to move quickly in front (on top) of the screen. The danger in using this defense is that the dribbler will gain the half step necessary to turn the corner and drive toward the basket. This momentary advantage is sometimes gained as the defensive player takes the short step up to move in front of the screener.

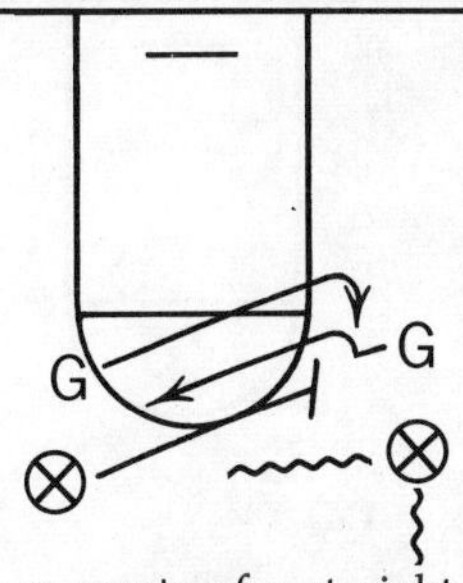

This is an example of a straight man-to-man defense with the defensive guard sliding behind the screen. This is the most popular method of handling this type of screening situation. The key to the success of this maneuver is that the defensive player guarding the screener must take a step backward to allow room for his defensive teammate to slide through.

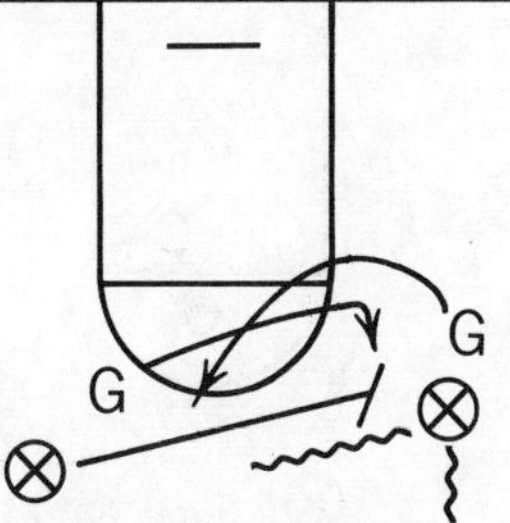

In this example, the defensive player guarding the dribbler goes behind both the screener and his defensive teammate. This situation is generally to be avoided because of the great distance to cover for the defensive player to catch up with the dribbler. This type of movement also gives the dribbler too much time to execute the jump shot after passing the screener.

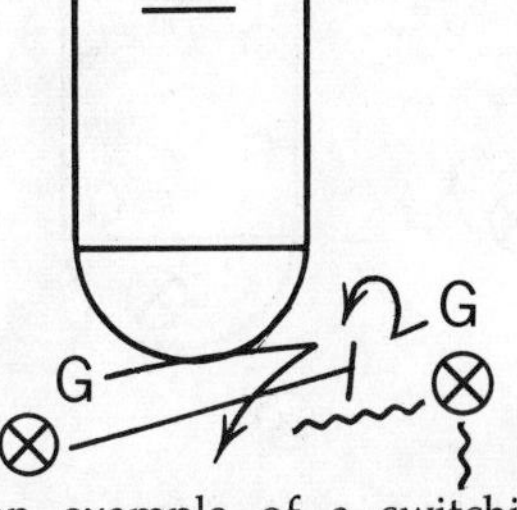

This is an example of a switching man-to-man defensive maneuver. There are two particularly important movements necessary for a successful switch to occur. The defensive player guarding the screener must step out quickly once he has decided to switch. The defensive player who is screened must quickly step backwards to take up a position behind the screener. If this is not done, the screener may be able to roll toward the basket and get a return pass from his teammate.

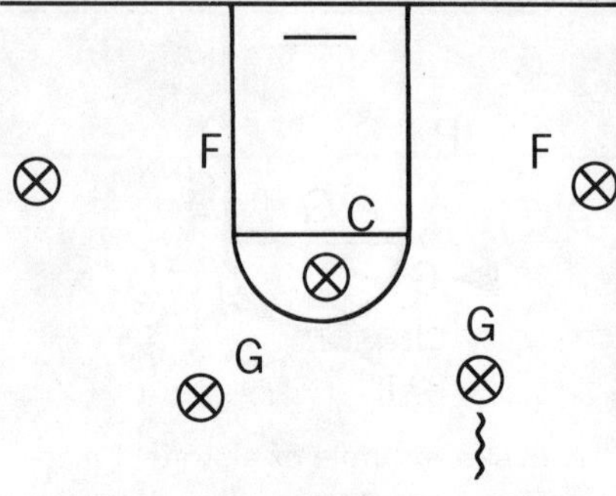

This is the straight man-to-man defensive alignment. Notice that each defensive player is almost playing his opponent "honestly." The weakside defensive forward has sagged slightly. The defensive center overplays his man slightly toward the strong side.

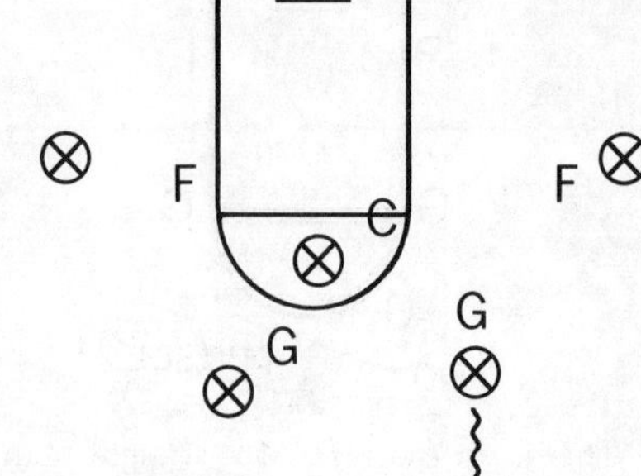

This is the very aggressive man-to-man defensive alignment. Notice that the offensive player with the ball has no clear passing lanes. Every defender is overplaying his man toward the ball. The defensive center is playing almost on the side of his man and should cut off the passing lane with his arms. The weakside defensive forward is away from his man, but he still has the passing lane effectively cut off.

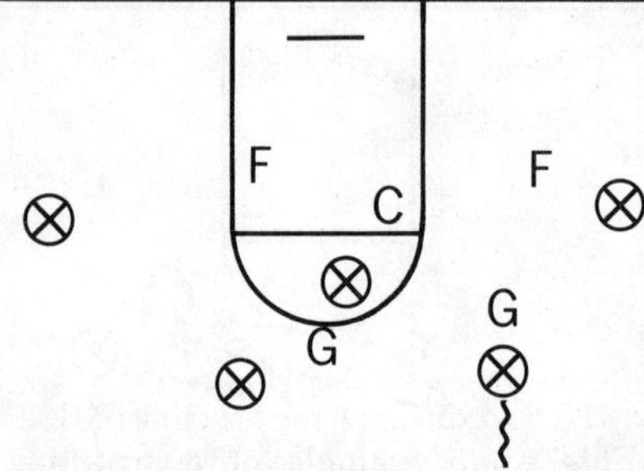

This is the sagging man-to-man defensive alignment. Notice that the weakside defensive guard and forward have both sagged toward the center scoring area. This defense is generally used against a high scoring pivot man.

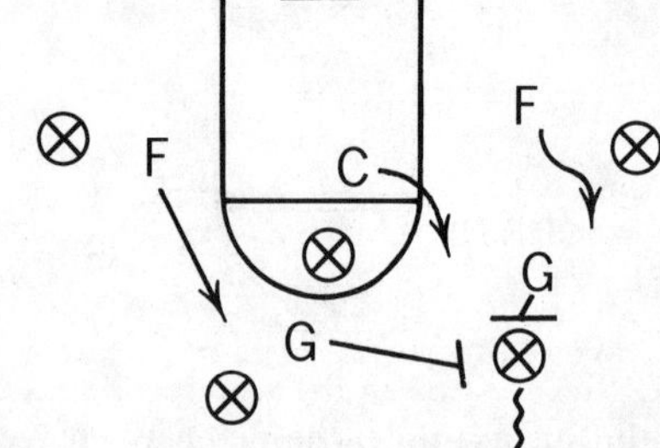

This is the trapping man-to-man defensive alignment. Notice that the weakside defensive guard has moved across to set the trap with the defensive player guarding the dribbler. When the trap is executed, the weakside defensive forward must move quickly up to be able to intercept a pass made to the weakside offensive guard. The defensive center and the strongside defensive forward move out to take away the passing lanes to their men.

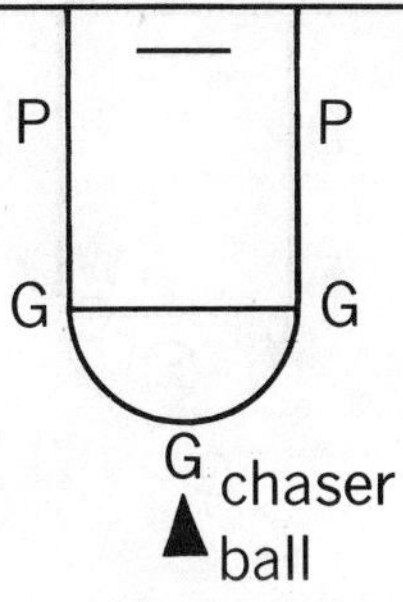

The four man box zone is used when the ball is directly in front of the basket. The chaser may either be a forward or a guard. An alternative to the use of the four man box zone is the four man diamond zone. The offensive point man can best be guarded in this situation by the use of a series of feints and jabs being made by the two defensive guards.

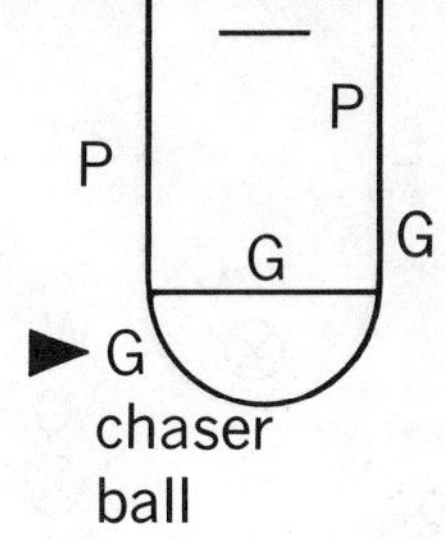

LG must defend against shots being taken from the territory he is in. LLP moves slightly out in anticipation of a pass being made down the side. RG moves down the center of the lane to block this passing lane.

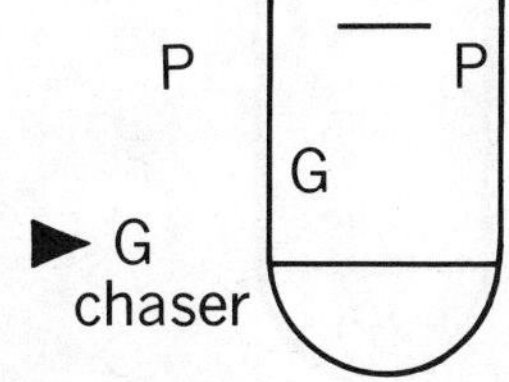

With the ball in the wing position LG must cover the territory where the ball is located as shown. Notice that RG has moved further down the center of the lane and RLP has stayed on the weak-side of the basket.

G
chaser P
P
G
G

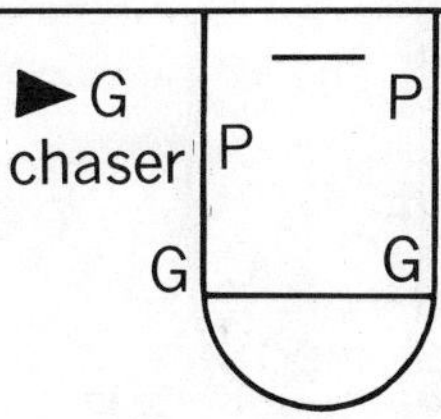

With the ball along the baseline the LLP must cover this territory. Notice that RG has moved all the way down to the strong side low position. This enables the taller and slower RLP to stay and rebound on the weak side of the basket.

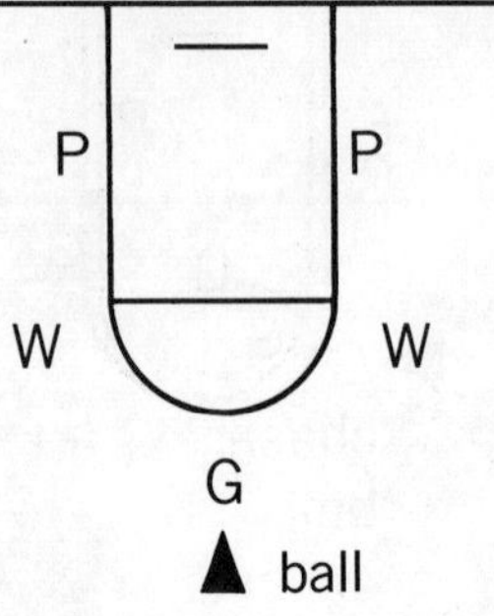

This type zone defense is not often used. This is probably due to the fact that it is vulnerable in the middle area, especially against an offensive high post player.

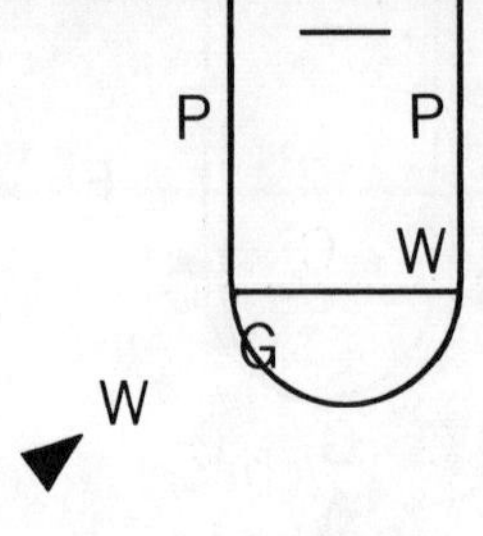

The greatest strength of this zone defense is that LW and RW are in excellent positions to cover the outside areas. In this case, RW and G have sagged into the middle to stop passes from being thrown to a high post man.

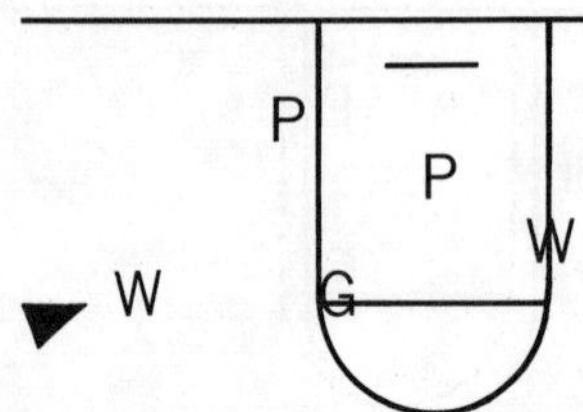

LW must also cover the territory where the ball is shown. RW and G have again sagged. RP has come across to plug up the middle area even more than usual. LP has begun to anticipate possible offensive threats being made along the left baseline.

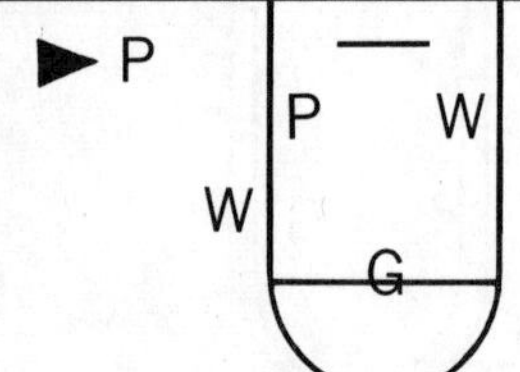

LP must cover the left baseline. RP moves across to cover the strong side low post and to do the strong side rebounding. RW moves down the lane to rebound on the weak side. LW and G sag to plug up the middle area.

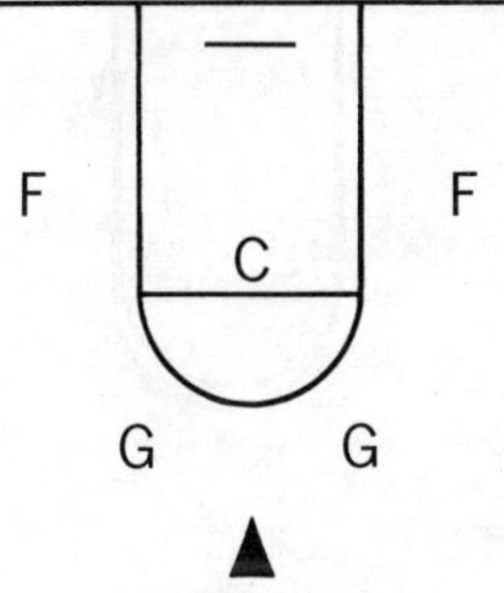

With the ball in front, this commonly used zone defense shows great strength. The difficulty that exists with the ball in this position is that the defense does not want to use both guards to stop the man with the ball. Some teams like to assign just one of the two guards to do this, and other teams prefer to have both guards use a series of feints to accomplish the task without having to fully commit themselves defensively.

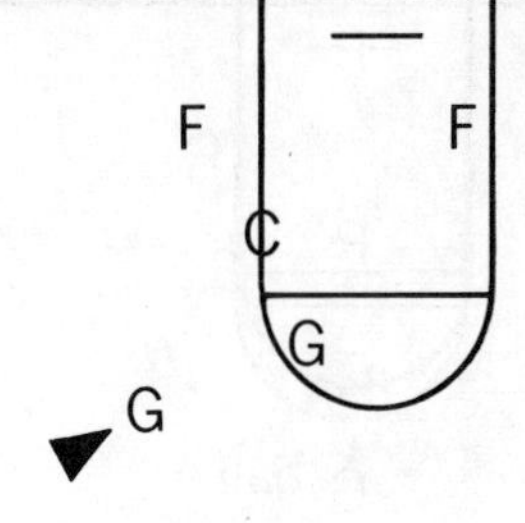

LG has the responsibility to stop offensive threats in this area. RF covers the weakside rebounding position. RG moves into the lane to prevent a pass from going to a high post player.

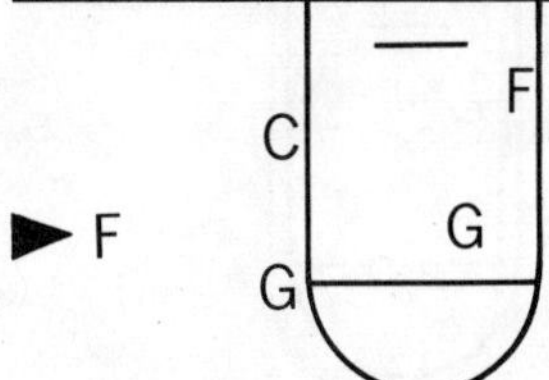

LF must cover the wing position in this defense. Notice that C has started his movement toward the baseline to cover a potential roving baseline player. RG has sagged even further into the lane.

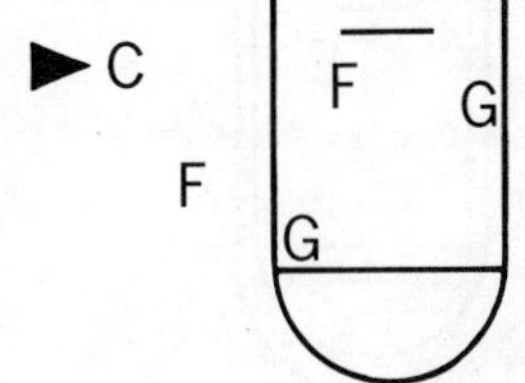

C must cover the baseline in this defense. He must anticipate passes being thrown in this area and be ready to move quickly to prevent the quick jump shot from being taken by the baseline player. RF has moved across the lane to cover the low post area. RG has moved down the right side of the lane to cover the weak side rebounding position.

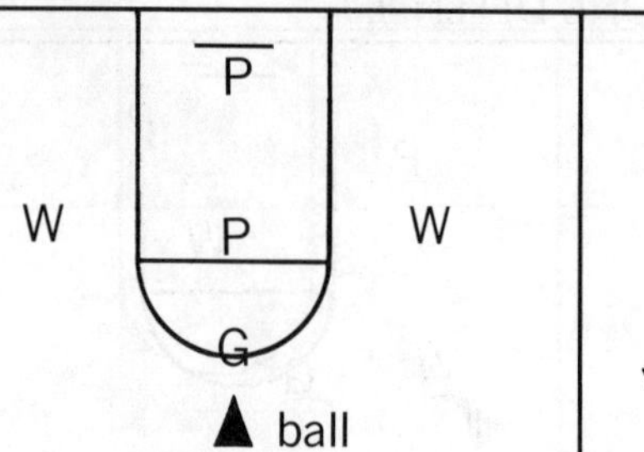

This zone is an especially strong one to use against a team that plays only one guard in front. The middle of the lane is well covered and so are the wings. The only apparent weakness in this formation is the baseline.

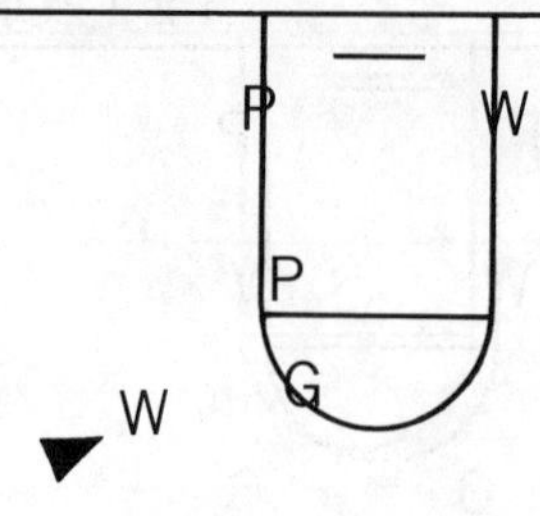

LW must cover offensive threats made in the area shown. RW moves back to the weakside rebounding position. LP patrols the baseline on the strong side.

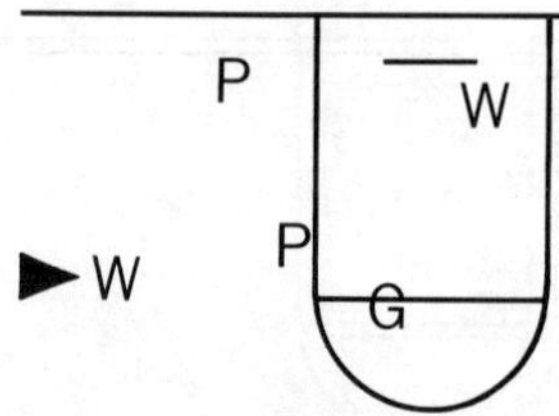

LW must also cover offensive threats made in the wing position. LP has moved further out on the baseline to cover a possible offensive threat being made in that area. G has sagged into the middle to help prevent passes from being made to a high post man.

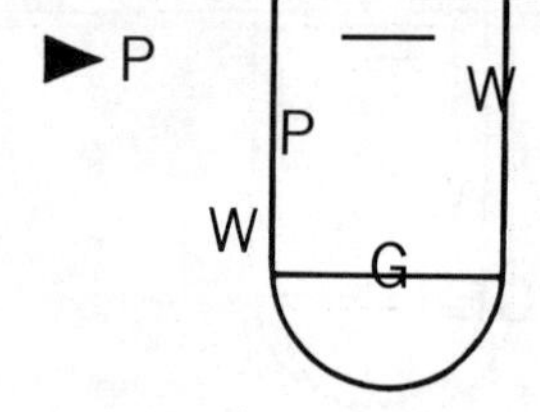

LP covers the baseline in this situation. RW has moved all the way back to cover the weak side rebounding position. LW and HP have sagged back to cover the middle area.

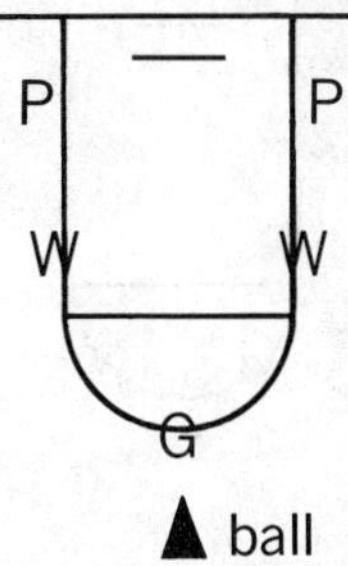

This popular zone defense has few weaknesses. Perhaps the most difficult task for the team using this zone is to cover the high post area adequately. If this can be done effectively, the defense is quite strong at all other positions.

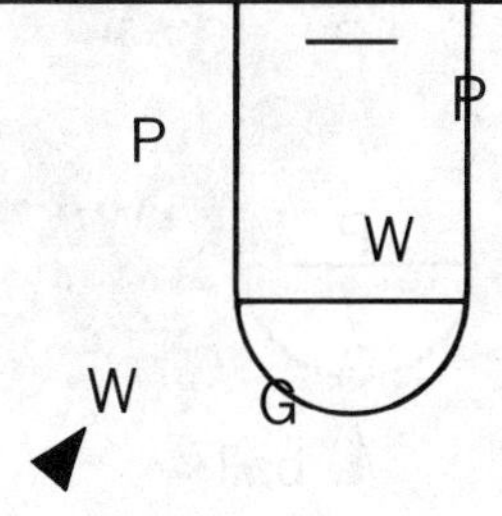

LW must cover the defensive area shown. RW has sagged into the middle to defend against an offensive high post player. G has sagged back into the middle for the same purpose.

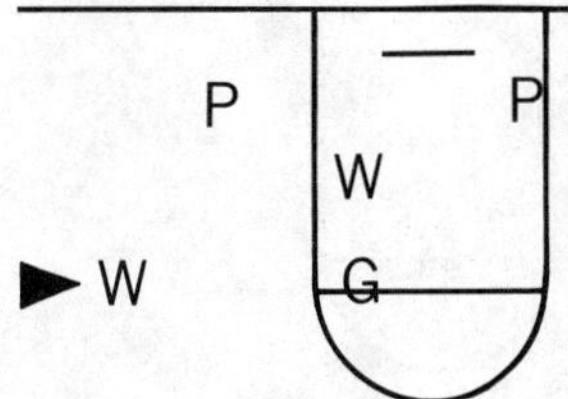

LW must also cover the area shown. RW and G again are primarily trying to cover the vulnerable middle area. LLP has begun to anticipate the possible offensive threats to be made along the left baseline area.

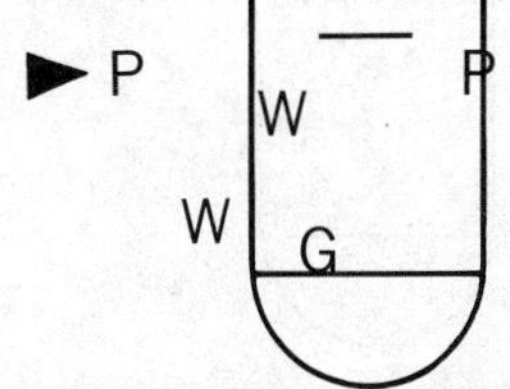

LLP covers the left baseline area. RW has come all the way across to cover the strong side low post. This leaves the larger and probably slower RLP to rebound on the weakside. LW and G sag to cover the middle area.

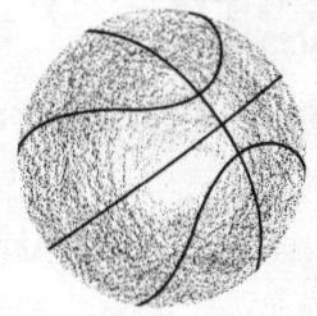

Selected Basketball Books

Anderson, Forrest and Albeck, Stan: *Coaching Better Basketball,* Ronald Press, New York, 1964, 259 pp.

Baisi, Neal: *Coaching the Zone and Man to Man Pressing Defenses,* Prentice-Hall, Inc., Englewood Cliffs, New Jersey, 1961, 190 pp.

Barnes, Mildred: *Women's Basketball,* Allyn and Bacon, Boston, 1972, 328 pp.

Bee, Clair: *The Science of Coaching,* A. S. Barnes, New York, 1942, 101 pp.

Brown, Lyle: *Offensive and Defensive Drills for Winning Basketball,* Prentice-Hall, Inc., Englewood Cliffs, New Jersey, 1965, 206 pp.

Carter, Ted: *Patterened Fastbreak Basketball,* Parker Publishing, West Nyack, New York, 1971, 219 pp.

Cousy, Robert and Power, Frank: *Basketball: Concepts and Techniques,* Allyn and Bacon, Boston, 1970, 500 pp.

Davis, Robert: *Aggressive Basketball,* Parker Publishing, West Nyack, 1969, 204 pp.

Dean, Everett: *Progressive Basketball,* Prentice-Hall, Inc., Englewood Cliffs, New Jersey, 1950, 271 pp.

Eaves, Joel: *Basketball's Shuffle Offense,* Prentice-Hall, Inc., Englewood Cliffs, New Jersey, 1960, 212 pp.

Esposito, Michael: *Game Situation Strategy in Basketball,* School-Aid Company, Danville, Illinois, 1960, 190 pp.

Harkins, Harry: *Tempo-Control Basketball,* Parker Publishing, West Nyack, New York, 1970, 218 pp.

Hobson, Howard: *Scientific Basketball,* Prentice-Hall, Inc., Englewood Cliffs, New Jersey, 1949, 250 pp.

Jucker, Ed: *Cincinnati Power Basketball,* Prentice-Hall, Inc., Englewood Cliffs, New Jersey, 1962, 172 pp.

Julian, Alvin F.: *Bread and Butter Basketball,* Prentice-Hall, Inc., Englewood Cliffs, New Jersey, 1960, 302 pp.

Loeffler, Ken: *Ken Loeffler on Basketball,* Prentice-Hall, Inc., Englewood Cliffs, New Jersey, 1955, 197 pp.

McCracken, Branch, *Indiana Basketball,* Prentice-Hall, Inc., Englewood Cliffs, New Jersey, 1955, 207 pp.

McGuire, Frank: *Team Basketball: Offense and Defense,* Prentice-Hall, Inc., Englewood Cliffs, New Jersey, 1966, 217 pp.

Neal, Patsy: *Basketball Techniques for Women,* Ronald Press, New York, 1966, 228 pp.

Newell, Pete, and Bennington, John: *Basketball Methods,* Ronald Press, New York, 1962, 350 pp.

Pinholster, Garland: *Encyclopedia of Basketball Drills,* Prentice-Hall, Inc., Englewood Cliffs, New Jersey, 1958, 228 pp.

Ramsay, Jack: *Pressure Basketball,* Prentice-Hall, Inc., Englewood Cliffs, New Jersey, 1963, 228 pp.

Rupp, Adolph: *Rupp's Championship Basketball,* Prentice-Hall, Inc., Englewood Cliffs, New Jersey, 1948, 239 pp.

Sharman, Bill: *Sharman on Basketball Shooting,* Prentice-Hall, Inc., Englewood Cliffs, New Jersey, 1965, 222 pp.

Strack, David: *Basketball,* Prentice-Hall, Inc., Englewood Cliffs, 1968, 612 pp.

Tarleton, Tom: *Tips and Ideas for Winning Basketball,* Prentice-Hall, Inc., Englewood Cliffs, New Jersey, 1965, 204 pp.

Wilkes, Glenn: *Basketball Coach's Complete Handbook,* Prentice-Hall, Inc., Englewood Cliffs, New Jersey, 1962, 306 pp.

Winter, Fred: *The Triple-Post Offense,* Prentice-Hall, Inc., Englewood Cliffs, New Jersey, 1962, 228 pp.

Wolfe, Herman: *From Tryouts to Championships,* Prentice-Hall, Inc., Englewood Cliffs, New Jersey, 1964, 205 pp.

Wooden, John: *Practical Modern Basketball,* Ronald Press, New York, 1966, 418 pp.

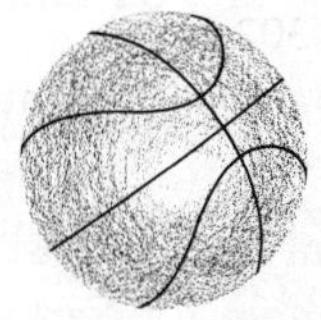

Selected Research Articles

Alley, L. B., and Maaske, P. M.: To Improve Shooting Accuracy, Practice at Small Baskets, *Athletic Journal, 42:*34, Sept., 1961.

Anderson, T.: Visual Aids in Shooting, *Research Quarterly, 13:*552, December, 1942.

Bell, T. B.: Training and Endurance, *Research Quarterly, 19:*229, October, 1948.

Bennett, C. L.: Relative Effectiveness of Four Activities in Developing Motor Ability, *Research Quarterly, 27:*253, October, 1956.

———: Effectiveness of Basketball in Developing Motor Abilities of College Women, *Research Quarterly, 27:*253, October, 1956.

Blake, R.: Distance Traversed by Basketball Players in Different Types of Defense, *Athletic Journal, 21:*18, January, 1941.

Boswell, C. H. and others: Is Basketball Too Strenuous? *Athletic Journal 19:*36, November, 1938.

Broer, M. R.: Reliability of Tests for Junior High School Girls, *Research Quarterly, 29:*139, May, 1958.

———: Effect of Basic Skills Instruction on Basketball Playing Ability, *Research Quarterly, 29:*379, December, 1958.

Buckley, C. W.: Mechanical Analysis of the Jump Shot, *Athletic Journal, 43:*8, October, 1962.

Bunn, J. W.: A Study of Baskets at Different Heights, *Athletic Journal, 13:*6, February, 1933.

———: The Standard Basketball for 1950–51, *Athletic Journal, 30:*32, November, 1949.

Burnham, Stan: Develop Your Rebounders With Weight Training, *Scholastic Coach, 30:*16, December, 1960.

Campbell, Donald: Heart rates of selected male college freshman during basketball season, *Research Quarterly, 39:*888, December, 1968.

Chui, E.: Effect of Weight Training on Jumping, *Research Quarterly, 21:*188, October, 1950.

Coleman, R. G.: Experiments in Basketball, *Athletic Journal, 10:*9, June, 1930.

Counts, John: Research on the Knox Basketball Test, unpublished master's thesis, The Ohio State University, 1963.

Cross, T. J.: Comparison of Whole and Part Methods of Learning Basketball, *Research Quarterly, 8:*49, December, 1937.

Dean, E. S.: Basketball Testing, *Athletic Journal, 27:*15, November, 1946.

Della, D. G.: Relation of Jumping to Foot Leverage, *Research Quarterly, 21:*11, March, 1950.

Di Giovanna, V.: Physical Measures Related to Success in Basketball, *Research Quarterly, 14:*203, May, 1943.

———: Basketball Ability and Posture, *Research Quarterly, 2:*74, May, 1931.

Dickinson, R. E.: Basketball Players at Work, *Scholastic Coach, 13:*25, December, 1943.

Edgren, H. D.: Basketball and Carry-Over Values, *Research Quarterly, 3:*159, March, 1932.

Elbel, E. R., and Allen, F. C.: Evaluating Basketball Performance, *Research Quarterly, 12:*538, October, 1941.

Fay, P. J., and Messersmith, L. L.: Effect of Rules Changes on Distances Traveled in Basketball, *Research Quarterly, 9:*136, May, 1938.

Fish, M. E.: Differences Between Two and Three-Court Game for Girls, *Research Quarterly, 9:*69, December, 1938.

Flanagan, L.: Personality of Participants in Basketball, *Research Quarterly, 22:*312, October, 1951.

Foti, J. C.: Does the 10-Second Rule Achieve Its Purpose? *Athletic Journal, 15:*15, March, 1935.

Frigard, W.: Effect of the Elimination of the Center Jump, *Research Quarterly, 10:*150, May, 1939.

Glassow, R. B., Colvin, V., and Schwartz, M. M.: Basketball Playing Ability of College Women, *Research Quarterly, 9:*60, December, 1938.

Harrison, Edward: A Test to Measure Basketball Ability for Boys, unpublisted master's thesis, University of Florida, 1969.

Hennis, G. M.: Basketball Knowledge Test for College Women, *Research Quarterly, 27:*301, October, 1956.

Hill, Elam R.: Basketball Coaches' Survey, *Scholastic Coach, 22:*18, October, 1952.

Hinton, E. A., and Rarick, L.: Basketball and Strength, *Research Quarterly, 11:*61, October, 1940.

———: Basketball and Vital Capacity, *Research Quarterly, 11:*61, October, 1940.

Hodgson, P.: Effect of Basketball on Physiological Functions, *Research Quarterly, 10:*53, October, 1939.

———: Physiological Reaction Following Basketball, *Research Quarterly, 7:*45, May, 1936.

———: Blood Pressure Following Basketball, *Research Quarterly, 7:*48, May, 1936.

Hosinki, John: An Investigation of the Use of Computer Assisted Instruction in Teaching the Shuffle Offense in Basketball, unpublished doctoral dissertation, Florida State University, 1965.

Humphrey, F.: Analysis of Team Efficiency, *Athletic Journal, 34:*42, November, 1953.

Kerr, Frances: An Investigation of the Relationship Between the Cardiac Cost During a Basketball Game and the Performance of Selected Basketball Skills, unpublished master's thesis, University of North Carolina at Greensboro, 1968.

LaPorte, W. R.: Time Allotment, *Research Quarterly, 7:*119, October, 1936.

Latchaw, M.: Basketball Wall Pass Test for the Elementary Grades, *Research Quarterly, 25:*439, December, 1954.

Lindeburg, F. A., and Hewitt, J. E.: Effect of Oversized Ball on Shooting and Ball Handling, *Research Quarterly, 36:*164, May, 1965.

Martie, J. E.: Effect of Basketball on Physical Development *Research Quarterly, 2:*86, May, 1931.

May, Carolyn: A Comparison of Three Basketball Free Throw Practice Situations: Effects on Accuracy Performance and Evidence of Ball Trajectory Transfer, unpublished master's thesis, University of Wisconsin, 1968.

McGee, R.: Attitudes Towards Competition for Girls, *Research Quarterly, 27:*60, March, 1956.

Messersmith, L. L., and Bucher, C. C.: Distance Traveled by Big Ten Players, *Research Quarterly, 10:*61, October, 1939.

Messersmith, L. L., and Corey, S. M.: Distance Traveled in Playing Basketball, *Research Quarterly, 2:*57, May, 1931.

Michael, E. D., and Gallon, A.: Effect of Training on the Circulation of Participants in Basketball, *Research Quarterly, 30:*303, October, 1959.

Miner, N., Hodgson, P., and Espenschale, A.: Time Spent in Activity, *Research Quarterly, 11:*94, March, 1940.

Mortimer, E. M.: Angle of Projection and Velocity in Basketball Shooting, *Research Quarterly, 22:*234, May, 1951.

Mullaney, D.: Free Throw Technique, *Athletic Journal, 38:*53, November, 1957.

Nelson, D. O.: Effects of Swimming and Basketball Upon Explosive Power, *Research Quarterly, 33:*581, December, 1962.

———: Transfer of Learning in Basketball, *Research Quarterly, 28*:364, December, 1957.

O'Connor, F., and Sills, F.: Heavy Resistance Exercises for Basketball Players, *Athletic Journal, 36*:6, June, 1956.

Olds, L. W.: Effect of Basketball on Physical Fitness, *Research Quarterly, 12*:254, May, 1941.

Olsen, E. A.: Relation of Psychological Capacities to Success in Basketball, *Research Quarterly, 27*:79, March, 1956.

Pacheco, B. A.: Effect of Warm Up on Jumping, *Research Quarterly, 30*:202, May, 1959.

Patrick, K.: Quick Reaction Time Means Athletic Ability, *Athletic Journal, 30*:68, September, 1949.

Peterson, H. D.: A Scientific Approach to Shooting in Basketball, *Athletic Journal, 40*:32, October, 1959.

Richardson, D. E.: The Shuttle Run as a Basketball Conditioner, *Athletic Journal, 38*:52, October, 1957.

Russell, N., and Lange, E.: Achievement Scales in Basketball, *Research Quarterly, 9*:43, December, 1938.

Saltis, L. R.: Accuracy in Basketball, *Athletic Journal, 23*:33, January, 1943.

Scanlon, William: A Study to Determine the Results of Focusing Attention on a Point of Reference in Basketball Field Goal Shooting, unpublished master's thesis, Springfield College, 1968.

Schaus, Fred: Time-Motion Study of Basketball Practice, *Scholastic Coach, 26*:7, December, 1956.

Schwartz, H.: Girl's Achievement Test, *Research Quarterly, 8*:152, March, 1937.

Scolnick, Anthony: An Electrogoniometric and Cinetographic Analysis of the Arm Action of Expert Basketball Jump Shooters, unpublished doctoral dissertation, Springfield College, 1967.

Scott, M. G., and Matthews, H.: Fatigue from Basketball, *Research Quarterly, 20*:138, May, 1949.

Singer, R. N.: Practice Effects on Acquisition and Retention of a Novel Skill, *Research Quarterly, 36*:68, March, 1965.

Snell, C.: Basketball Knowledge Tests, *Research Quarterly, 7*:79, March, 1936. Also, *8*:153, March, 1937.

Stroup, F.: Relation of Playing Ability to Peripheral Vision, *Research Quarterly, 28*:72, March, 1957.

———: Validation of a Skills Test, *Research Quarterly, 26*:353, October, 1955.

Swegan, D., and Thompson, H. L.: Effects of Warm-Up in Swimming and Basketball, *Scholastic Coach, 27*:20, November, 1957.

Thompson, C. W., Buskirk, E. R., and Goldman, R. F.: Changes in Weight and Body Fat of Players, *Research Quarterly, 27*:418, December, 1956.

Thompson, H.: Effect of Warm-up on Basketball, *Research Quarterly, 29*:231, May, 1958.

Tisdale, H.: Value of Therapeutic Program in Physical Fitness, *Research Quarterly, 5*:56, October, 1934.

Tussing, L.: Effect of Basketball on Vision, *Research Quarterly, 11*:16, March, 1940.

Vroom, G. A., and Nixon, K. E.: Fundamental Basketball Skills of College Freshmen, *Athletic Journal, 36*:16, March, 1956.

Wakefield, M. C.: Longevity of Basketball Players, *Research Quarterly, 15*:2, March, 1944.

Wellesley College Studies in Hygiene and Physical Education, Analysis of Frequency of Occurrence of Technical Elements in Basketball, *Research Quarterly, 9*:67, March, 1938, Supplement.

Wilden, P. P.: Comparison of Two Methods of Teaching Basketball, *Research Quarterly, 27*:235, May, 1956.

Zimmerman, H. M.: Jumping Differences in Skilled and Non-Skilled Performers, *Research Quarterly, 27*:352, October, 1956.

Index